GW00720749

£12.30

Systematic Course Design for the Health Fields

Systematic Course Design for the Health Fields

ASCHER J. SEGALL, M.D.

HANNELORE VANDERSCHMIDT

RUANNE BURGLASS

THOMAS FROSTMAN

Prepared by the CENTER FOR EDUCATIONAL DEVELOPMENT IN HEALTH
(*formerly the* TEACHER PREPARATION PROGRAM)

HARVARD SCHOOL OF PUBLIC HEALTH

A WILEY BIOMEDICAL—HEALTH PUBLICATION

JOHN WILEY & SONS, INC., *New York* ● *London* ● *Sydney* ● *Toronto*

This project was supported by grant number 5D04AH01049-04, awarded by the Division of Associated Health Professions, Bureau of Health Manpower, Department of H.E.W., and by contract number AID/csd-3613, awarded by the Technical Assistance Branch, Agency for International Development, Department of State.

Copyright © 1975, by John Wiley & Sons, Inc.

All rights reserved. Published simultaneously in Canada.

No part of this book may be reproduced by any means,
nor transmitted, nor translated into a machine
language without the written permission of the publisher.

Library of Congress Cataloging in Publication Data:

Main entry under title:

Systematic course design for the health fields.

    (A Wiley biomedical-health publication)
    Includes bibliographies and index.
    1. Medicine—Study and teaching. 2. Para-medical
education. I. Segall, Ascher J. II. Harvard University.
School of Public Health. Teacher Preparation Program.
[DNLM: 1. Public health—Education. WA18 H339s]
R834.S95   375'.61   75-20398
ISBN 0-471-77410-3

Printed in the United States of America

10 9 8 7 6 5 4 3 2 1

Preface

This book forms the framework for a course on systematic curriculum design that has been offered at the Harvard School of Public Health for the past five years. The purpose of the book is twofold:

1. To be used as the basic text for courses on curriculum design in the health fields, both in the United States and in the developing world.
2. To be used as a guide to course design efforts by teachers working by themselves or as a team.

The Course Design Model

We present a particular systematic approach for developing courses that are relevant to the future professional needs of the students. We refer to this approach as our "course design model."

This model has been evolved over a five-year period with successive versions revised not only on the basis of specific comments and suggestions but also on the basis of students efforts to apply the model to courses that they were designing.

The final version has three major phases, each of which is composed of two or more "Tasks," as follows:

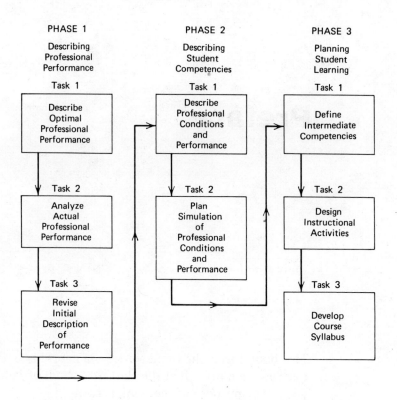

PHASE 1
Describing Professional Performance

Task 1
Describe Optimal Professional Performance

Task 2
Analyze Actual Professional Performance

Task 3
Revise Initial Description of Performance

PHASE 2
Describing Student Competencies

Task 1
Describe Professional Conditions and Performance

Task 2
Plan Simulation of Professional Conditions and Performance

PHASE 3
Planning Student Learning

Task 1
Define Intermediate Competencies

Task 2
Design Instructional Activities

Task 3
Develop Course Syllabus

Since the course design model forms the structural basis for this book, it will be helpful from time to time to refer to this diagram.

Structure of Materials

This book is divided into four major units:

Unit A   Overview of the Course Design Model
Unit B   Implementation Problems
Unit C   Methods to Facilitate Application
Unit D   Supplements

Unit A, as its title implies, is intended merely to *overview* the procedures and concepts involved in the model. Here we simplify the details of implementing the model and provide only those examples that are necessary to clarify the basic processes. Each of the three chapters in Unit A are devoted to one of the three phases of the model.

Unit B is intended primarily for those who are actually trying to implement the course design model. The three chapters in Unit B (again one for each phase of the model) are organized around specific *problems* that teachers often encounter when they apply the model to their own instructional situations. For each problem identified, materials are provided that demonstrate the nature of the problem and, at least, one way of solving it.

Unit C describes alternative methods and techniques that are often used in the implementation of various aspects of the course design model. Each method is discussed briefly and is followed by an indication of its advantages and limitations. When appropriate, annotated bibliographies are provided for those who wish a more detailed presentation.

Unit D includes a complete guidance system, that is step-by-step guidelines for performing each task in the course design model. It also contains a complete example that demonstrates the products suggested by the guidance system. Finally, an index refers the reader to definitions of technical terms, examples, and passages where important concepts are used or developed.

How to Use This Book

Since we intend this book as a "handbook," we have tried to design it for easy reference use. However, we urge readers to become familiar with the general flow of the model and basic terminology by scanning Unit A before they attempt to utilize the other units. In Unit B, one could work through all the "mini-cases" and practice exercises in a systematic fashion, or could read only those sections that deal with problems actually being encountered during the design of a course. These materials are self-instructional but also can be the basis for class exercises or small group discussions. Readers are encouraged to scan the contents of Unit C and then to read sections more carefully when they are needed or referred to in other parts of the text.

Acknowledgements

Primary thanks are due to the hundreds of students who have worked with these materials during the last several years. Their suggestions and criticism were invaluable in writing and organizing the book, and portions of their student projects have been adapted for use as examples and mini-cases throughout the text.

Teaching Assistants for I.D. 202 and 203, Teaching Preventive Medicine and Public Health and Curriculum Design, made a substantial contribution. In teaching with these materials, they were able to identify problem areas and generously gave their time for review of their concerns and suggestions.

Teaching Assistants include:

Dr. Kamal Abou-Daoud	Mr. Thomas Frostman	Dr. Kenneth Rothman
Dr. Bethania Aller	Ms. Carlie Goodwin	Dr. Steven Silberman
Ms. Carolyn Arnold	Dr. Charles Hays	Ms. Norma Swenson
Dr. William Bird	Dr. Grace Kleinbach	Dr. Hannu Vuori
Dr. Milton Burglass	Dr. Steven Marlowe	
Dr. Catherine De Angelis	Dr. Elliott Miller	
Dr. Dodge Fernald		

Special mention must be given to Dr. Catherine De Angelis whose student project formed the basis of the "Pediatric Paramedical Care" example, which is used throughout Unit A and is pulled together in Unit D as a continuous example of each developmental stage.

Particular thanks are also due to Teaching Fellows who participated in this program. They used the material to prepare their own course designs, taught others with the materials, and helped develop examples. Two of the Fellows, Dr. Theodore Bell and Dr. Dodge Fernald, made valuable contributions to sections of the book.

Substantive contributions were made by the following leaders in the field of educational technology whose work has formed the basis for much of the development of these materials.

Abt Associates, Inc.

Dr. Coleman Bender, Professor of Organizational Communication, Emerson College

Dr. Donald Bullock, Director, The Center for Educational Technology, Catholic University of America

Mr. Joseph Harless, President, Harless Performance Guild, Inc.

Mr. Robert Horn, President, Information Resources, Inc.

Dr. Robert Mager, President, Mager Associates

Dr. Douglas Porter, Harvard Medical School

Dr. Frederick Pula, Director, University Audio-Visual Services, Boston College

Dr. Kay Stolurow, Health Science Center, State University of New York at Stonybrooke

We also thank those individuals who are directing the field testing of *Systematic Course Design for the Health Fields* in five developing countries during 1974 to 1976. They include:

Dr. Jaime Arias	Asociacion Colombiana De Facultades De Medicina	Bogota, Columbia
Mr. Le Khac Dien	Ministry of Health	Saigon, Vietnam
Dr. Dodge Fernald	Harvard School of Public Health	Boston, Massachusetts
Dr. Jorge Haddad	University of Honduras	Tegucigalpa, Honduras
Dr. Lazare Kaptue	Centre Universitaire Des Sciences De La Sante	Yaounde, Cameroun
Dr. Dieter Koch-Weser	Harvard Medical School	Boston, Massachusetts
Dr. Duong Trong Thieu	Ministry of Health	Saigon, Vietnam
Dr. Francisco Yepes	Asociacion Colombiana De Facultades De Medicina	Botota, Columbia

The enthusiastic support of our editor Earl Shepherd and the Wiley staff are also greatly appreciated. And finally, we are grateful to Ms. Ruth Pettis, staff assistant and librarian, who assumed bibliographical control and developed the index; to Ms. Geri Higgins, staff assistant, who typed and formated the field test edition of the book; and to Ms. Ramona Arnett, who assumed administrative direction.

BOSTON, MASSACHUSETTS

SEPTEMBER, 1975

Ascher J. Segall

Hannelore Vanderschmidt

Ruanne Burglass

Thomas Frostman

Contents Summary

Contents

CHAPTER 3 OVERVIEW OF
Phase 3: Planning Student Learning

UNIT B   Implementation Problems

CHAPTER 4 IMPLEMENTATION PROBLEMS RELATED TO
Phase 1: Describing Professional Performance

UNIT C   Methods to Facilitate Application   C-1

CHAPTER 7   METHODS FOR

Phase 1: Describing Professional Performance   C-5

CHAPTER 8   METHODS FOR

Phase 2: Describing Student Competencies   C-29

CHAPTER 9 METHODS FOR
Phase 3: Planning Student Learning

UNIT D Supplements

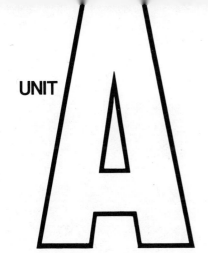

Overview of the Course Design Model

Unit A

OVERVIEW OF THE COURSE DESIGN MODEL

INTRODUCTION

Unit A describes a three-phase model for designing courses. It proposes a systematic approach for developing courses that are relevant to the future professional needs of the students.

Each of the three chapters in Unit A is devoted to one of the three phases of the course design model. These three phases are:

1. Describing professional performance.
2. Describing student competencies.
3. Planning student learning.

Unit A is intended merely to **overview** the procedures and concepts involved in the course design model. An attempt is made to simplify the details of implementing the model and to provide only those examples deemed necessary to clarify the basic processes.

Chapter 1

OVERVIEW OF PHASE 1: DESCRIBING PROFESSIONAL PERFORMANCE

Contents

INTRODUCTION

"Another two-hour lecture on statistical measures of signifi-cance! Why do I have to know all that?

What does all this have to do with being a physician? How will I use statistics in my clinical work?"

How can one develop courses that are relevant to the needs of the students?

A visiting professor responsible for teaching medical students "Statistical Methods Applied to Medicine" might begin by requesting last year's syllabus or a list of topics he is expected to cover. An inexperienced instructor might prefer to begin by discussing with more experienced colleagues how they approach course development.

Still other approaches could involve reviewing lecture notes taken in related college courses, scanning available textbooks, or asking students what they are interested in.

Although any of these approaches might lead to a course that is "interesting" and "well received," there is no guarantee that any of them will result in learning which is **relevant** to the future needs of the students . . ., that is, learning which will facilitate effective performance by these students in their subsequent professional roles.

To develop instruction that will be relevant to student needs, one must begin with an analysis of those student needs. That is, one must identify:

(a) the professional roles students will assume after completing their training.

(b) what constitutes effective performance within these roles.

Depending on the scope of the course being developed, the professional performance to be analyzed may involve all aspects of the future roles, or only those aspects that are related to a more narrowly defined content area, such as pathology or biostatistics. In either case, once this professional performance has been identified, it can serve as the basis for relevant course objectives, and instruction can then be designed to prepare students for their future roles in the health fields.

Thus the key to guaranteeing that a course will be relevant to student needs is the identification of future professional performance. For this reason, "describing professional performance" is the first phase of the systematic course design model.

CHAPTER PURPOSE

The purpose of this chapter is to describe and demonstrate each of the major tasks involved in describing professional performance that is both idealistic and realistic. These tasks are:

1. To describe the **optimal** professional performance.
2. To analyze the **actual** professional performance.
3. To revise the initial description on the basis of discrepancies between optimal and actual professional performance.

DESCRIBING THE INSTRUCTIONAL SITUATION

However, even before one is ready to begin the tasks of Phase 1, it is important to have a clear picture of the **instructional situation** within which the course is being prepared.

DEFINITION

> ## INSTRUCTIONAL SITUATION
>
> – The context or framework within which the course is to be developed and taught.
>
> – May include:
>
> *Title* – official or temporary name for course
>
> *Purpose(s)* – major intent of the course
>
> *Students* – major category(s) of individuals who will take the course (e.g., third year medical students, community volunteers, etc)
>
> *Setting* – institution or location where the course will be taught
>
> *Resources* – funds, personnel, labs, and audiovisual aids, etc. available to develop and teach course
>
> *Constraints* – limiting factors such as time schedules, numbers of students, or traditions which must be maintained

Taking a few minutes to describe the above elements of the instructional situation not only gives the instructor perspective on the course to be developed, but also facilitates communication with colleagues regarding the course.

EXAMPLE

The instructional situation described below is the basis for examples of each aspect of the course design model, as described throughout Chapters 1 to 3. All of these examples are brought together as one continuous example in Chapter 11.

INSTRUCTIONAL SITUATION

Title: Pediatric Paramedical Care

Purpose: To enable participants to care for the needs of pediatric patients presenting with the most common complaints encountered in an outpatient setting, either

(a) by providing treatment themselves, or
(b) by referring the case to a physician and arranging ancillary data collection if appropriate.

Students: Registered nurses with at least two years of nursing experience, who have elected to become paramedics

Setting: Lashley University Medical Center in New York City

Resources: Sufficient funds are available to cover the costs of all necessary materials including reprints, slides, videotapes, and the like. The instructor is available to spend full-time on this course. Other full-time instructors, pediatric residents and interns, a pediatric nutritionist, and a social worker could be made available for short periods of time, but not for major teaching responsibilities. Classrooms are fully equipped with audiovisual equipment, and outpatient examining rooms are available for labs at least one day a week. A well equipped lab where routine urine and hematology work can be performed is also accessible.

Constraints: Course begins in six months and must conform to dates established by the regular school semester at Lashley University. This schedule allows for two 2-hour class sessions and one 3-hour lab period each week for 30 weeks, or a total of 210 class hours for the year. For each class hour, students can be expected to spend between 1 and 2 hours outside of class working on assignments. Up to 20 students will take the course each year, and they must be prepared to pass certification requirements by the end of the year.

TASK 1:

Describe Optimal Professional Performance

OVERVIEW

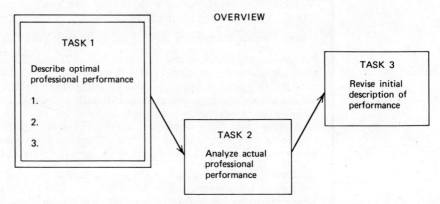

The first task involved in "describing professional performance" is to describe the optimal performance of practitioners in the future professional settings of the students. Note that initially we are concerned with specifying **optimal** professional performance, which is not necessarily identical with current practices.

DEFINITION

OPTIMAL **Professional Performance**

– **Performance of a professional practitioner that represents the most desirable or satisfactory execution of the responsibilities associated with that professional role.**

Tasks 2 and 3 of this first phase of the course design model are concerned with **actual** professional practices and their implications for the final description of professional performance. This final description will then be used in later stages to derive instructional objectives which define the competencies that students will be expected to acquire in the academic setting.

Describing optimal professional performance involves three steps:

1. Identifying future professional roles of the students,
2. Listing the professional responsibilities involved in these roles, and
3. Analyzing the skill, knowledge, and attitude components of each of these professional responsibilities.

Each of these steps in Task 1 are explained and demonstrated in the material that follows.

Describe
Optimal Pro-
fessional
Performance:

2. List profes-
   sional
   responsi-
   bilities
3. Analyze
   skill, knowl-
   edge, and at-
   titude com-
   ponents.

1. Identify Future Professional Roles

Before one can begin describing any performance, one must know **whose** performance is to be described. Thus the first step in describing optimal professional performance is to identify the future **professional roles** of the students.

DEFINITIONS

> **PROFESSIONAL ROLES**
>
> — The future positions, professions, occupations, or titles to be assumed by the students and for which the training is designed.
>
> — Ideally, the identification of future professional roles includes information about the setting in which the roles will be assumed.

EXAMPLES

Examples of professional roles:

- flight medical officers in an operational air force flying squadron
- directors of public health programs in the tropics
- pediatric nurses in well equipped American hospitals and clinics
- physicians practicing preventive medicine in rural areas of Saudi Arabia
- volunteer community health workers in rural areas of California

It is important to include information about the professional setting since in many ways the setting determines **how** the responsibilities of a professional role can be executed. For example, the process of diagnosing illness is somewhat different for physicians practicing in urban America where the most advanced laboratory technology is available than for physicians practicing in rural areas of lesser developed countries where many diagnostic tests are not available. Consequently the training needs for these two groups of physicians differ somewhat, and this difference should be reflected in the descriptions of professional performance for the two roles.

CROSS-REFERENCE

If the future professional roles of your students are widely divergent or unknown, consult the guidelines provided in Problem 1 of Unit B, page B-6.

Describe
Optimal Pro-
fessional
Performance:

1. Identify fu-
   ture profes-
   sional roles

3. Analyze
   skill, knowl-
   edge, and at-
   titude com-
   ponents

2. List Professional Responsibilities

Having established the roles for which students are being prepared, the instructor next identifies the **professional responsibilities** associated with these roles as related to the scope of the course.

DEFINITION

> **PROFESSIONAL RESPONSIBILITIES**
>
> — **Activities for which students will be accountable in their future professional roles.**
>
> — **Duties or tasks performed by a competent practitioner in a professional role.**

EXAMPLES

Professional responsibilities may involve such activities as:

    (a) performing an operation
    (b) making a decision
    (c) following a procedure
    (d) collecting information
    (e) evaluating an activity

Note the specification of responsibilities in "action" terms. This early emphasis on "behaviors" allows the instructor ultimately to design a course that will focus on developing student skills rather than "increasing knowledge of . . ." or "increasing understanding of . . ." or "instilling an appreciation for. . . ."

Though "knowledge," "understanding," and "appreciation" are essential in carrying out the responsibilities, it is the **application** of these elements by which professional performance is judged, and it is the **application** for which the training will be designed.

NON-EXAMPLES

Accordingly, the following do **not** constitute "professional responsibilities:

    (a) **knowing** facts or procedures about . . .
    (b) **understanding** concepts or theories to . . .
    (c) **having** an **appreciation** for . . .
    (d) **being aware** of . . .

GUIDELINES FOR LISTING RE-SPONSIBILITIES

1. Each statement of professional responsibility should:

    (a) represent optimal professional performance, and
    (b) be related to the scope and purpose of the course.

2. It is usually advisable to organize the list of responsibilities:

    (a) according to the order of their performance, and/or
    (b) into a series of functional categories.

COMPLETE EXAMPLES   Below are listed the professional responsibilities for two different roles.

CROSS-REFERENCES   For additional examples and guidelines on how to identify professional responsibilities for difficult instructional situations, see Problems 2 and 3 in Unit B, beginning on page B-12.

LIST OF PROFESSIONAL RESPONSIBILITIES
(Course Title: Pediatric Paramedical Care)

A pediatric paramedic (in urban America):

1. Takes a complete medical history from parent when appropriate.

2. Performs a complete pediatric physical examination when appropriate.

3. Performs abbreviated physical exams when needed.

4. Performs or arranges for pertinent laboratory and diagnostic tests.

5. Refers child to physician if necessary, providing appropriate clinical notes as well as test findings.

6. Provides treatment and follow-up care for each of the following types of problems:

    a. Gastroenteritis (vomiting, diarrhea, etc.)
    b. Simple acute upper respiratory infections (e.g., colds, otitis media, pharyngitis, etc.)
    c. Simple dermatitis (impetigo, mild eczema, acne, etc.)
    d. Most nutritional problems (obesity, feeding problems, etc.)
    e. Immunizations

7. Provides the ongoing health educational aspects of the following types of problems (in conjunction with physician care):

    a. Behavior problems (e.g., enuresis, hyperactivity, sleep phobia, thumb sucking, etc.)
    b. Chronic diseases (e.g., diabetes mellitus, asthma, etc.)
    c. Adolescent problems (e.g., pregnancy, V.D., drugs, etc.)

8. Arranges for social service referrals if appropriate (e.g. for cases of child battery, lead poisoning, etc).

9. Maintains clinical records in a problem-oriented fashion.

LIST OF PROFESSIONAL RESPONSIBILITIES
(Course Title: Nutritional Surveillance)

District Medical Officers (in rural East Africa):

A. **Regarding problem analysis**

    1. Assess the adequacy of existing dietary, agricultural, and medical records for communities in their districts.
    2. Initiate new data collection systems if required to provide needed baseline data.
    3. Identify categories of local population at greatest risk.
    4. Determine nature and extent of existing malnutrition.
    5. Evaluate community and medical resources for treatment and prevention.

B. **Regarding problem solution**

    1. Design feasible treatment and prevention systems.
    2. Develop plans for implementing their systems.
    3. Train staff to establish components of their systems.
    4. Supervise ongoing operation of their systems.

Describe
Optimal Pro-
fessional
Performance:

1. Identify fu-
   ture profes-
   sional roles.
2. List profes-
   sional
   responsi-
   bilities

3. Analyze Skill, Knowledge and Attitude Components

The professional responsibilities identified by the instructor will serve as the basis for communication between that instructor and professionals currently practicing in the specified role(s). Such a dialogue provides useful information regarding **actual** professional performance.

Before this dialogue occurs, however, the course designer should clarify the meaning of each responsibility by describing its components. That is, for each responsibility identified, the following questions should be asked: When a competent practitioner executes this responsibility:

(a) what **skills** are involved?
(b) what **knowledge** is necessary?
(c) what **attitudes** are desirable?

DEFINITIONS

SKILLS

- Steps required to execute a professional responsibility.

- Cognitive and motor procedures involved in performing the activity described by a professional responsibility.

KNOWLEDGE

- Concepts, facts, criteria for decisions and other cognitive aspects of a responsibility.

- Information required to execute a skill component or the responsibility as a whole.

ATTITUDES

- Values, feelings, sentiments and other affective aspects of a responsibility.

- General style or approach toward others, oneself, or one's work which facilitate execution of a skill component or the responsibility as a whole.

The next page displays the analysis of the first responsibility for a pediatric paramedic (as listed on page A-13).

ANALYZED RESPONSIBILITY

Responsibility No. 1: Takes a complete medical history from parent when appropriate.

SKILLS	KNOWLEDGE	ATTITUDES
1. Recognizes when a complete history is necessary. 2. Puts parent and patient at ease.	– Complete history necessary in initial, nonemergency visit. – Factors often making patients uncomfortable and ways to avoid them.	– Sympathetic to discomfort of the patient.
3. Determines history details using directed but nonleading questions: **Chief complaint** including age (accurate in months), race, and sex.	– Difference between leading and nonleading questions, and between directed and nondirected questions.	– Desire to make medical history nonthreatening to parent.
Present illness including signs and symptoms, and duration of each.	– General meaning of various signs and symptoms, and other signs and symptoms associated with each.	
Birth history including birth weight; age, gravity, parity and abortions of mother; length of gestation; neonatal problems and feeding habits.	– Definitions of gravity, parity, abortion, gestation, neonatal problems to watch for.	– Senses importance of thoroughness and accuracy in taking histories.
Past history including previous hospitalizations, serious accidents or illnesses, communicable diseases, immunizations, and developmental milestones.	– Standard immunization routine. – Common communicable diseases. – Normal neonatal developmental milestones.	– Is honest in recording even those statements from parents which appear contradictory or irrelevant.
Family history including three generations whenever possible, and general health of each member.	– Method for plotting family tree by age, appropriate illness, and deaths.	
Social history including type of house, number of people living in house, occupation of parents, nature of parents' relationship to child.		
Review of systems including respiratory otolaryngeal, cardiovascular, gastrointestinal, genito-urinary, endocrine, neurologic, and bones-joints-muscles.	– Specific questions to ask related to each system.	
4. Records history details on history form.	– Appropriate formats for each type of history data.	– Strives for legibility, clarity, and completeness when recording history details.

The instructor includes in this analysis **only** those skills, knowledge, and attitudes that are **essential** in executing the responsibility. For in describing these components of the responsibility the designer not only is establishing a basis for communication with others, but also is identifying the substantive elements to be covered in the course. Nonessential elements could cloud communication and could introduce irrelevant subject matter into the instruction.

CROSS-REFERENCES

For additional examples and guidelines on how to analyze skill, knowledge, and attitude components, see Problems 4 and 5 in Unit B, beginning on page B-26.

For convenience and future reference, the product of Task 1 (i.e., describe optimal professional performance) will be referred to as the **initial mastery description**.

DEFINITIONS

MASTERY DESCRIPTION

- **The complete *set* of analyzed responsibilities.**

- **The description of a competent practitioner or "master performer" in a specified professional role.**

INITIAL MASTERY DESCRIPTION

- **The product of describing *optimal* professional performance before analyzing *actual* professional performance.**

- **The initial listing of professional responsibilities and component skills, knowledge, and attitudes.**

INTRODUCTION TO THE GUIDANCE SYSTEM

After each major task of the course design model has been described and illustrated, the steps, procedures, and products involved in that task will be summarized as on the following page for Task 1 of Phase 1. These summaries are titled "guidance system," since they are designed to guide your application of the course design model by serving as a checklist-review. The full guidance system is compiled as one continuous unit in Chapter 10, beginning on page D-5.

GUIDANCE SYSTEM

PHASE 1: DESCRIBING PROFESSIONAL PERFORMANCE

Task 1: Describe Optimal Professional Performance

STEPS	PROCEDURES	PRODUCTS
1. Identify the future professional roles of the students.	a. Indicate the future positions or titles to be assumed by students and for which training is designed. b. If future roles are widely divergent or unknown, review Problem 1 beginning on page B-6.	A phrase describing the future role(s) of the students, including information about the setting or environment in which they will practice.
2. List professional responsibilities associated with the future roles.	a. Identify the activities, duties or tasks of competent practitioners in the role(s) identified. Each activity should: — represent optimal professional performance, and — be related to the scope and purpose of the course. b. If you have difficulty with this step, consult Problems 2 and 3 in Unit B, beginning on page B-12.	A list of responsibilities for each role, organized sequentially and/or by meaningful categories.
3. Analyze the skill, knowledge, and attitude components of each responsibility.	For each responsibility: a. identify the **skills** or steps required to execute that responsibility b. list information the practitioner must **know** or be aware of to execute a skill component or the responsibility as a whole, and c. indicate **attitudes** practitioners should have towards others, themselves, or their work to facilitate execution of a skill component or the responsibility as a whole. If you have difficulty with this step, consult Problems 4 and 5 in Unit B, beginning on page B-26.	*Initial mastery description: The complete set of professional responsibilities analyzed in terms of skill, knowledge, and attitude components. Alternative formats for these analyzed responsibilities are shown on the next page.

*Needed in subsequent steps of the course design model.

SUGGESTED FORMATS

(For Each Analyzed Responsibility
in the Mastery Description)

Course Title: _____

ANALYZED RESPONSIBILITY

Responsibility No. ___ : _____

SKILLS	KNOWLEDGE	ATTITUDES
1. ____	____	____
2. ____	____	____
3. ____	____	____

(OR)

Course Title: _____

ANALYZED RESPONSIBILITY

Responsibility No. ___ : _____

A. SKILLS:
   1. _____
   2. _____
   3. _____

B. KNOWLEDGE
   1. _____
   2. _____
   3. _____

C. ATTITUDES
   1. _____
   2. _____

TASK 2:

Analyze Actual Professional Performance

OVERVIEW

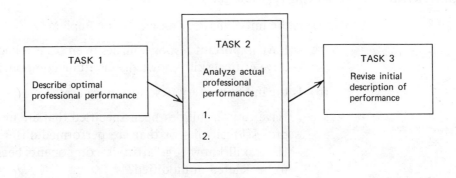

TASK 1

Describe optimal professional performance

TASK 2

Analyze actual professional performance

1.

2.

TASK 3

Revise initial description of performance

*"If I've specified in detail the **optimal** performance of my students as professionals, why should I also analyze what people are actually **now doing** in those roles?*

*I'm not concerned with what **they are doing** . . . I just want to make sure my students perform as well as possible."*

The product of Task 1 is an initial mastery description, that is, a listing of the course-relevant professional responsibilities for the future professional roles of the students, and a specification of the skill/knowledge/attitude components associated with each responsibility.

Producing an initial mastery description is a crucial step toward ensuring that course objectives reflect the performance requirements of professional roles. What is necessary next is to analyze **actual** professional performance to verify the initial mastery description so that overlooked responsibilities can be added to the initial descriptions and inappropriate responsibilities can be deleted or modified.

DEFINITION

> **ACTUAL PROFESSIONAL PERFORMANCE**
>
> — Practices currently associated with a given professional role, as determined by appropriate method(s) of performance analysis.
>
> — Data related to the actual performance that can be expected of students in the future.

EXAMPLE

A young instructor was developing an advanced course in epidemiology. After carefully describing the responsibilities of a professional epidemiologist, the instructor discussed his list with a group of experts (experienced professional epidemiologists).

It soon became clear that an important element in the epidemiologist's profession had been omitted from the instructor's list, namely, his involvement in activities of a management nature.

The experts agreed that epidemiologists must spend a significant amount of time and effort "promoting," that is, obtaining grant money, defending proposals for research, campaigning for facilities and human resources, etc. They felt that an epidemiologist's training was clearly incomplete if it failed to prepare students for these activities.

IMPORTANT QUESTIONS	In analyzing actual professional performance, it is useful to consider the following types of questions:

(a) Is the initial mastery description **complete**?

  – Have important responsibilities been overlooked?
  – Have critical skill/knowledge/attitude components been ignored?

(b) Is the initial mastery description **accurate**?

  – Have responsibilities been specified that are not appropriate for the professional roles or that are performed differently than expected?
  – Have skill/knowledge/attitude components been included that need to be deleted or modified?

(c) Are actual practitioners performing **competently**?

  – Are certain responsibilities performed poorly?
  – Are any skill/knowledge/attitude components giving practitioners particular difficulty?

To answer the above questions, and thus to analyze actual professional performance, one must:

(1) select and implement a method for analyzing actual professional performance, and
(2) identify discrepancies between optimal and actual performance.

Each of these steps in Task 2 are explained and demonstrated below.

Analyze
Actual Profes-
sional Perfor-
mance:

2. Identify
   perfor-
   mance dis-
   crepancies.

1. Select and Implement a Method of Performance Analysis

The first step in analyzing actual professional performance is selecting a method of performance analysis which will:

(a) allow one to assess what practitioners are doing, what they are not doing, and what they are not doing well; and

(b) be feasible to implement in terms of such developmental constraints as time, money, and personnel.

DEFINITION

> **PERFORMANCE ANALYSIS**
>
> — The collecting of information concerning actual professional performance.
>
> — The verification of an initial mastery description through an analysis of actual professional performance.

METHODS OF PERFORMANCE ANALYSIS

Most methods of performance analysis involve one or more of the following specific techniques:

1. **QUESTIONNAIRE.** Obtaining information about job conditions and responsibilities through written responses to a series of questions.

2. **CRITICAL INCIDENT TECHNIQUE.** Collecting reports of key personal experiences with effective and ineffective performance on the part of practicing professionals.

3. **LOG DIARY.** Having practitioners describe their activities throughout specified work periods.

4. **CHECKLIST.** An exhaustive list of task statements that can be used by a worker or an observer to verify which of the tasks are actually part of the job.

5. **OBSERVATION INTERVIEW.** Interviewing one or more practitioners at the work site **while** they are performing.

6. **WORK PARTICIPATION.** Involves the direct work performance by the **investigator**, with or without guidance from experienced professionals.

7. **INDIVIDUAL INTERVIEW.** Interviewing one or more professionals about their practice (generally away from the work environment).

8. **GROUP INTERVIEW.** Interviewing a group of professionals or experts in the specified professional field.

9. **TECHNICAL CONFERENCE**. A group of subject matter experts collectively determine the responsibilities of the position under investigation.

CROSS-REFERENCES	For more detailed descriptions and references for the above methods of performance analysis, consult Unit C beginning on page C-3.

For consideration of how to choose among the various methods of performance analysis, see Problem 6 in Unit B beginning on page B-51. If the future role does not currently exist, see Problem 7, page B-56.

EXAMPLE

In the case of the young instructor developing an advanced course in epidemiology (page A-19), a major discrepancy between the initial description of professional performance and actual professional performance was discovered through an informal group interview. Clearly, this was an efficient and inexpensive approach that yielded valuable information regarding the future role of the students . . . information that could lead to changes in the instructor's thinking and in the course itself.

Another method of performance analysis that the instructor might have used is the questionnaire. Information regarding the activities of an epidemiologist could be obtained from a large number of professionals by asking them either to write answers in their own words to open-ended questions, or to select answers from specific alternatives. Compared to the informal group interview technique, the questionnaire approach is more costly and time consuming, but it can be distributed to a broad range of practitioners, resulting in a larger data base to compare information from various categories of respondents.

"But what if I don't have time to do a performance analysis?"

Resource and time constraints may make it impractical for an instructor to carry out an extensive performance analysis. In this respect, two considerations are worth noting:

(a) Every effort should be made to verify the initial mastery description to ensure that it does relate to the realities of actual professional performance. Many times even a single interview or visit with a practitioner will reveal significant information about actual professional performance.

(b) Even if the course developer cannot analyze actual professional performance, basing course objectives on initial mastery description increases significantly the likelihood that these course objectives will be reasonably relevant to students' needs in their future professional work.

Analyze Actual
Professional Per-
formance

1. Select method
   of perfor-
   mance analysis

2. Identify Performance Discrepancies

Once the method(s) of performance analysis have been implemented and data are available regarding actual professional performance, the next step is to identify *performance discrepancies* between the initial mastery description and actual professional performance. These may lead to revision of the initial mastery description.

DEFINITION

PERFORMANCE DISCREPANCIES

— A "mismatch" between the initial mastery description and actual professional performance. That is:

(a) Responsibilities or components specified in the initial mastery description which in actual practice are

— performed differently
— *not* performed well, or
— *not* performed at all.

(b) responsibilities or components which are performed in actual practice but were *omitted* from the initial mastery description.

EXAMPLE

A course is being developed to train medical assistants to perform immunizations in rural health centers in developing countries. Included in the initial mastery description are the following responsibilities:

— Identifies those individuals within their areas who need immunizations.
— Keeps systematic records of immunizations.
— Prepares summary reports for district medical officers.

After observing the operations of the health centers and discussing the immunization work with incumbent assistants and district medical officers, the instructor located the following discrepancies:

(1) Medical assistants do keep records of immunizations, but generally not in a systematic fashion.
(2) They do **not** prepare and submit reports to district medical officers, at least not very often.

The next section describes how to revise the initial mastery description on the basis of an analysis of the **causes** of the performance discrepancies.

First, however, there is a review of the major steps for Task 2, analyzing actual professional performance.

GUIDANCE SYSTEM

PHASE 1: DESCRIBING PROFESSIONAL PERFORMANCE

Task 2: Analyze Actual Professional Performance

STEPS	PROCEDURES	PRODUCTS
1. Select and implement method(s) of performance analysis.	a. Review methods of performance analysis in Chapter 7, beginning on page C-5 and guidelines for selection on page C-55. b. Consider feasibility of implementation in view of constraints such as the availability of: – time – money – practitioners or other subject matter experts, and – resources needed to analyze data. c. Plan and carry out performance analysis.	Instruments used in the performance analysis, such as: – questionnaires – checklists – questions for interviews – audiotapes for recording technical conferences.
2. Identify performance discrepancies.	a. Compare findings of performance analysis with initial mastery description. b. Look for: –responsibilities or components specified in initial mastery description which in actual practice are · performed differently · not performed well, or · not performed at all – responsibilities or components which are performed in actual practice but were omitted from initial mastery description.	*List of performance discrepancies.

*Needed in subsequent steps of the course design model.

TASK 3:

Revise Initial Description of Performance

OVERVIEW

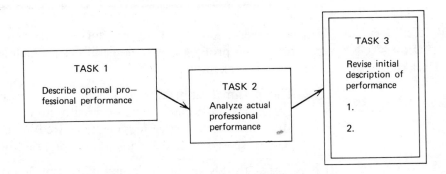

"Originally I had planned to train medical assistants to prepare summary reports for the district officers. In practice, however, they do not do this. Should I include this responsibility in my final mastery description or not?"

Having specified **optimal** performance and analyzed **actual** performance, the instructor is ready to develop a more definitive version of the mastery description by asking:

(a) Should missing responsibilities or components (not initially specified) be added to the mastery description?

(b) Should unconfirmed responsibilities or components (not verified in practice) be discarded?

(c) Should responsibilities or components that are implemented differently in actual practice be modified?

To answer these questions, the instructor first determines the **reasons** for the discrepancies between the initial mastery description and actual performance. That is:

— Why are practitioners performing differently than expected? Is there a new or better way?

— Why are they **not** performing a particular responsibility or component skill well?

— Why are they **not** performing certain responsibilities at all? Should they be?

— Why are they performing unanticipated responsibilities? Were they merely overlooked in the initial mastery description or do they represent departures from more traditional professional practices?

Asking questions like these raises the issue of performance standards, that is, the issue of what the professionals in a particular role really **ought** to be doing, as opposed to what they are **in fact** doing or what the instructor originally **thought** they should do.

DEFINITION

PERFORMANCE STANDARDS

— Criteria for judging or evaluating the acceptibility or quality of performance.

— A basis for determining what the professional performance *ought* to be.

SOURCES OF PERFORMANCE STANDARDS

There are several sources of performance standards that can be used in determining which professional responsibilities to include in the final mastery description. For example:

(a) The personal subjective judgments of the instructor, perhaps supported by informal discussions with other subject matter experts.

(b) More formal, objective judgments arrived at through consensus data, that is, the combined judgments of qualified persons.

If one wishes to rely on more formal consensus-determined standards, then the performance analysis should include items and questions designed to elicit suitable information from a large number of qualified respondents. This may complicate the performance analysis effort, but also does provide some assurance that final decisions about the revised mastery description will reflet a consensus of the experts.

Task 3 (Revising the initial description of performance) involves two steps:

1. Analyzing the causes of performance discrepancies which have been identified.

2. Modifying the initial mastery description.

The remainder of this chapter further explains and illustrates each of these steps.

<table>
<tr><td>

Revise the
Initial Descrip-
tion of Perfor-
mance.

2. Modify the
mastery
description

</td></tr>
</table>

1. Analyze the Causes of Performance Discrepancies

Resolving certain performance discrepancies may present little difficulty. For example, a responsibility or component may simply have been overlooked during the initial specification of mastery; or once the actual professional situation is observed, it may be evident that incumbent practitioners have found a "better" way of carrying out a certain responsibility.

However, other discrepancies may be more complex, and resolving them may require additional analysis. For example, you may discover that professionals are **not** doing something which in fact they should be doing, or that they are not doing something well. Most of these more complex performance discrepancies can be attributed to:

(a) a lack of *skills* or *knowledge* on the part of the incumbents,
(b) inhibiting *attitudes* (or lack of facilitating attitudes), and/or
(c) inhibiting *environmental* factors.

Finding answers to the following types of questions may prove helpful in identifying the factors responsible for a specific performance discrepancy:

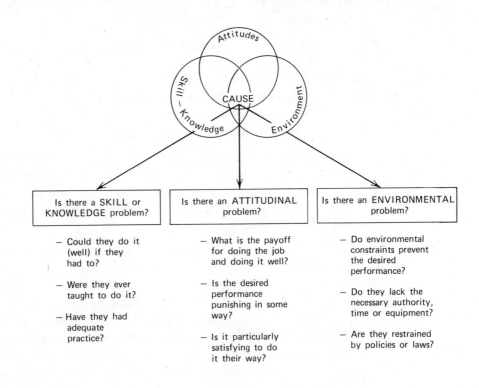

Is there a SKILL or KNOWLEDGE problem?	Is there an ATTITUDINAL problem?	Is there an ENVIRONMENTAL problem?
— Could they do it (well) if they had to? — Were they ever taught to do it? — Have they had adequate practice?	— What is the payoff for doing the job and doing it well? — Is the desired performance punishing in some way? — Is it particularly satisfying to do it their way?	— Do environmental constraints prevent the desired performance? — Do they lack the necessary authority, time or equipment? — Are they restrained by policies or laws?

EXAMPLE   In the previous medical assistant example (page A-23) one performance discrepancy identified was related to inadequate record-keeping of immunizations. In analyzing the cause(s) of this performance problem, the instructor discovered that medical assistants had never been taught a systematic method for keeping records (lack of skill/knowledge) and, hence, that they were "playing it by ear," doing just enough paper work to "get by."

He also discovered that they basically **wanted** to do a good job, so if they knew how to keep good records, they probably would do so (i.e., no attitudinal problems identified).

Finally, the medical assistants had the time, facilities, and authority to keep such records and, therefore, environmental factors could not be blamed for the lack of good record-keeping.

Noting that the main cause of the performance deficiency seemed to be a lack of skills and knowledge, the instructor retained the responsibility relating to record-keeping in the mastery description and decided to emphasize systematic procedures for keeping records.

However, in the same performance analysis, another unconfirmed responsibility was identified:

"Prepares monthly reports for district medical officers."

In analyzing the causes of this performance discrepancy, the instructor found that

(1) Medical assistants **did** in fact know how to prepare the reports, or at least this was not the major problem.
(2) Preparing reports was both time-consuming and boring; medical assistants did not like to prepare reports.
(3) They never received feedback from their district medical officers and were not encouraged to send in the reports.

The instructor concluded that this was an attitudinal problem attributed primarily to environmental factors. In discussing the situation with several district medical officers, he found they rarely read the reports when they did receive them and, in general, did not consider these reports particularly important.

The best solution to this type of problem may be administrative rather than educational. Perhaps an entirely new reporting system is needed; or perhaps the district officers need training in how to identify potential problems by charting progress. However, the instructor may not be in a position to influence administrative decisions, but nonetheless must train the medical assistants. In such a case, the best solution would be to emphasize the importance of regular reporting by illustrating the types of problems that can be uncovered in this way but, at the same time, to warn students that, at present, their supervising officers may not be using or even reading the progress reports.

Revise the
Initial Descrip-
tion of Perfor-
mance

1. Analyze
   causes of
   perfor-
   mance dis-
   crepancies

2. Modify the Initial Mastery Description

As noted previously, the *purpose* of analyzing the causes of performance problems is to help the course designer decide:

(a) whether **instruction** is an appropriate solution to the problem;
(b) how the mastery description should be revised to describe the substantive basis for such training.

After analyzing the cause of each performance discrepancy, the instructor should:

(a) add missing responsibilities and components if they were left out of the initial mastery description by oversight and are now deemed appropriate.
(b) discard unconfirmed responsibilities or components if they are **not** necessary in the actual professional role.
(c) modify responsibilities or components if different or better ways of discharging these responsibilities are identified.

EXAMPLE

The initial mastery description for a hospital lab technician included the responsibility: "Cleans and sterilizes all utensils and equipment." The performance analysis for this role revealed that as a rule lab technicians do **not** clean or sterilize equipment because this is done by lab assistants. Therefore, this responsibility was discarded from the revised mastery description.

However, it was also discovered that the lab technicians **were** responsible for training and supervising their own lab assistants in this and other supporting tasks. Thus, two new responsibilities were added to the initial mastery descriptions as follows:

(a) trains lab assistants to clean and sterilize utensils and equipment.
(b) supervises quality of lab assistant's work.

GUIDELINES

1. Whenever the decision is made to **add** new responsibilities or components to the initial mastery description, these new responsibilities or components must be **relevant** to the purpose and scope of the course.

2. Instructional constraints such as time and facilities must also be considered. Many times it is simply **not** possible to teach everything that theoretically should be taught. Decisions about the relative importance of the different professional responsibilities can help guide final decisions about what is retained in the final description of mastery performance, which will then serve as a basis for course objectives.

CROSS-REFERENCE

For a continuous example that illustrates both Task 2 (analyzing actual professional performance) and Task 3 (revising the initial description of performance), see Problem 8 in Unit B, beginning on page B-62.

GUIDANCE SYSTEM

PHASE 1: DESCRIBING PROFESSIONAL PERFORMANCE

Task 3: Revise the Initial Description of Performance

STEPS	PROCEDURES	PRODUCTS

1. Analyze causes of performance discrepancies.	Determine to what extent each discrepancy can be attributed to
	
	   — skill/knowledge factors
	   — attitudinal factors
	   — environmental factors.
		Explanations for each performance discrepancy

2. Modify initial mastery description.	If a discrepancy is attributed primarily to: Then consider:
	
	Skill/knowledge → Adding or
	  factors emphasizing a
	             responsibility or
	             appropriate skill/
	             knowledge components
	
	Attitudinal → Adding or
	  factors emphasizing an
	            attitude component to appropriate responsibilities
	
	Environmental → Discarding the responsibility or component, or
	  factors
	
	            Retaining the responsibility but adding environmental constraints as knowledge components.
		*Revised mastery description, which may be either
		
		— the initial mastery description which has been changed by additions, subtractions, and modifications,
		         or
		— a totally new mastery description.

*Needed in subsequent steps of the course design model.

WHERE ARE WE? Revising the initial mastery description completes the tasks of Phase 1 (DESCRIBING PROFESSIONAL PERFORMANCE). At this point, the instructor has produced a document that is referred to as the **revised mastery description.**

DEFINITION

> **REVISED MASTERY DESCRIPTION**
>
> — The final product of Phase 1 of the course design model.
>
> — A delineation of the responsibilities of a competent practitioner in the future professional role of the students, which:
>
>   (a) is limited to those responsibilities that are pertinent to the purpose and scope of the course,
>
>   (b) includes specification of the skills, knowledge, and attitudes which compose each responsibility, and
>
>   (c) represents a modification of optimal performance based on an analysis of actual performance.

Theoretically, acquiring the capabilities represented by this revised mastery description is a long-range professional goal for students in the course being designed. Therefore, basing objectives for the course on this mastery description assures that the instruction will be relevant to the future professional needs of the students.

The next chapter describes how to derive course objectives from a revised mastery description.

Chapter 2

OVERVIEW OF PHASE 2: DESCRIBING STUDENT COMPETENCIES

Contents

INTRODUCTION

*"One of the responsibil-
ities which my public
health students will
assume as professional
epidemiologists is to
determine when an
epidemic exists.*

*Can acquisition of this
ability represent an
objective for my
course?*

*Surely this activity is
much too complex for
a student! So many
factors could influence
such a determination!"*

The revised mastery description represents the performance of **competent** professionals. As such it reflects not only their formal academic training but also the refinement of their skills over time through actual experience. Often it is not realistic to expect students to attain the same level of competence as described in the mastery description.

Thus in deriving course objectives from the mastery description, it may be necessary to consider teaching students to approximate or simulate certain aspects of the professional performance. For example, for the professional responsibility of arranging follow-up care for patients under treatment, the derived course objective might involve preparing plans for the follow-up care of patients described in case studies.

The extent to which course objectives can approximate actual professional performance depends to a large extent on questions of feasibility. Given a specific time period (e.g., one semester), students with certain entering qualifications, and limited resources, how closely can students be expected to simulate the professional performance of mastery by the end of the course?

Phase 2 of the course design model addresses this problem; specifically, it deals with the determination of end-of-instruction course objectives, based on and derived from the revised mastery description. These course objectives will be called the **terminal student competencies.**

DEFINITION

TERMINAL STUDENT COMPETENCY

— **Capability or expertise expected of students at the end of and as a result of the instructional experience.**

— **May be specified at the level of professional competence or at some level approximating (i.e., simulating) professional competence.**

EXAMPLES

Professional Responsibility	*Terminal Student Competency*
Administer cardiopulmonary resuscitation to a person in need.	Administer cardiopulmonary resuscitation to a mannequin.
Assess the adequacy of existing dietary, agricultural, and medical records for communities in their districts.	Describe (a) procedures for determining the nature of existing dietary, agricultural, and medical records in a community, and (b) criteria for determining whether or not such records are adequate.

CHAPTER PURPOSE

The purpose of this chapter is to outline a method for describing competencies expected of students at the end of a course which are:

(a) based on the professional performance specified in the revised mastery description, and

(b) feasible to attain and assess during the instructional process.

There are two major tasks involved in describing terminal student competencies:

1. To describe professional competencies in terms of conditions and performance.
2. To plan the simulation of professional conditions and performance at levels appropriate to the instructional situation.

SELECTING RESPONSIBIL- ITIES FOR INCLUSION IN THE COURSE

It should be noted at the outset that it may not be feasible (or desirable) to derive terminal student competencies from **every** responsibility in the mastery description. Often time contraints prevent the consideration of all aspects of the mastery performance, even at low levels of simulation. And sometimes a responsibility may be too advanced or too trivial to merit instructional effort in a particular course.

Therefore, when deriving terminal student competencies for the course to be designed, the teacher should first select from the mastery description those responsibilities on which it is feasible to focus the instruction.

Describe
Terminal
Student Com-
petencies

2. Plan simu-
   lation of
   profes-
   sional con-
   ditions and
   perfor-
   mance

1. Describe Professional Conditions and Performance

The first task in describing a terminal student competency to be acquired during instruction is to specify the conditions and performance involved in the professional competency. That is, for each responsibility in the mastery description for which instruction will be developed, the instructor specifies:

(a) Typical **conditions** under which the students eventually will be expected to perform as professionals.

(b) The **performance** of a competent practitioner discharging; the responsibility under those conditions.

DEFINITION

> ## CONDITIONS
>
> — **The set of circumstances under which performance occurs.**
>
> — **Significant aspects of the environment that influence the expected behavior(s) involved in a competency.**

Conditions may include:

(a) other people, (clients, patients, other health professionals, etc).

(b) resources and facilities (money, equipment, and space).

(c) a problem, challenge, or task (to be solved, met, or executed).

(d) physical location (geographic, urban-rural, etc).

(e) physical stress (especially extremes, e.g., of temperature, sound, and elevation).

(f) time constraints (for completing a task).

(g) emotional stress (such as emergency situations, political pressures, etc).

DEFINITION

> ## PERFORMANCE
>
> — **Behavior(s) executed in the presence of specified conditions.**
>
> — **Behavior(s) indicating satisfactory demonstration of a competency.**

The specification of professional performance may include criteria such as:

(a) accuracy requirements (how precisely?)

(b) completeness requirements (how thoroughly?)

(c) rate/time requirements (how quickly?)

(d) safety requirements (avoiding/minimizing what risks?)

EXAMPLE   The first responsibility in the mastery description for a pediatric paramedic (see pages A-15) is:

"Takes a complete medical history from parents
when appropriate."

Typical **conditions** under which a practicing pediatric paramedic executes this responsibility include:

— a clinical setting
— access to a variety of pediatric cases
— forms for recording histories
— access to aids such as decision flowcharts for major complaints, questions pertinent to each organ system, etc.

Typical **performance** of a competent pediatric paramedic under the above conditions includes:

— deciding whether a complete history is needed,
— putting the patient and parent at ease,
— taking the medical histories and
— recording the data on the history forms:

In the above example, notice that the **performance** is a summarized version of the skill components of the responsibility as analyzed on page A-15.

The goal of the instructor is to **replicate** the professional conditions and performance whenever possible either by

(a) **recreating the professional environment in the classroom** (e.g., by bringing patients into the classroom for students to take medical histories), or by

(b) **moving the classroom to the professional setting** (e.g., by having students take medical histories under supervision in an out-patient clinic).

However, even when it is not possible to **replicate** the conditions and performance of a professional responsibility during instruction, the course designer still may be able to **approximate** the professional setting at a fairly high level of simulation.

Describe Terminal Student Competencies

1. Describe professional conditions and performance

DEFINITION

2. Plan Simulation of Professional Conditions and Performance

Having specified the conditions and performance characterizing the professional competency, the next step for the course designer is to determine the **level of simulation** that will characterize the terminal student competency (the level of simulation for the end-of-instruction course objective).

LEVEL OF SIMULATION

— The degree to which both the *conditions* of the instructional setting and the required student *performance* approximate the conditions and performance of the professional setting.

Often instructional constraints preclude replication of professional conditions and performance. In this event the conditions and/or performance associated with the professional setting must be modified so that achievement of the terminal student competency:

(a) is feasible within the limitations of the instructional setting, and
(b) can be assessed at the end of instruction.

EXAMPLE

The instructor of the course on pediatric paramedical care did not consider it feasible to replicate all the professional conditions and performance associated with the first responsibility in her mastery description. Therefore, she modified the specifications in a series of small steps to arrive at the highest level of simulation that she considered feasible for the course (see worksheet on page A-38).

PROFESSIONAL AND TERMINAL STUDENT COMPETENCIES

Responsibility No. 1: Takes a complete medical history from parent when appropriate.

CONDITIONS	PERFORMANCE
Professional Competency: When given a variety of pediatric cases in a clinical setting, history forms, and any needed decision guides . . .	. . . practitioners determine when complete medical histories are needed, put patients and parents at ease, take histories, and record data on history forms.
Terminal Student Competency: 1. When given *a typical* pediatric case in a clinical setting, history forms, and any needed decision guides . . .	. . . students will put the patient and parent at ease, take a medical history, and record the data on a history form.
2. When given *the instructor* playing the role of a parent with a sick child, in a clinical setting, with history forms and any needed decision guides . . .	. . . students will put the "parent" at ease, take a medical history, and record the data on the history form.
3. When given *a fellow student* who has been primed with a patient scenario in a classroom setting, a history form and any needed decision guides . . .	. . . students will put the "parent" at ease, take a medical history, and record the data on the history form.

(handwritten margin notes:)
Typical for the Professional setting
Not considered feasible for this Course
Highest level of simulation feasible for this Course

Notice that the main differences in levels of simulation for this example are in the **conditions**. With the exception of "determine when complete medical histories are needed" (which is present only in the professional competency), the same basic performance occurs at each level.

CROSS-REFERENCE

For additional examples and guidelines on how to derive terminal student competencies form professional responsibilities, see Problem 9 in Unit B, beginning on page B-70.

In the example on page A-40, why were levels #1 and #2 not considered feasible for the highest level of simulation?

Several limiting factors affect the degree to which the instructor can simulate the professional conditions and performance, including:

CONSTRAINTS ON SIMULATION

(a) *Students' Entry Competencies.* Previous level of learning which limits the ultimate performance that can be expected during instruction, given the time allocated for the instruction.

(b) *Simulation Resources.* Time, money, facilities, and personnel limiting the ability to replicate professional conditions and performance.

(c) *Implications of Formal Testing.* Type of evaluation needed, affecting how the terminal student competencies can be assessed.

Each of these limiting factors is explained in more detail in the remainder of this chapter.

Describe Terminal Student Competencies

1. Describe professional conditions and performance.

2. Plan simulation of professional conditions and performance, taking into consideration:

    b. Resources for simulation
    c. Needs for evaluation

a. Entry Competencies

One factor that limits the final level of simulation feasible for a course is the degree of competence with which students enter the course.

Most instruction operates within definite time limits. For example, a course may have allocated to it three hours per week for one semester. Thus, the amount of learning that can occur is limited by the course time constraints. The more relevant the background students bring into the course, the more feasible is their progression toward higher levels of simulation of professional competencies. It is in this context that the entry competencies of students can be a factor limiting the level of simulation at which the terminal student competencies are set.

It is useful for the instructor to examine his students' previous academic and professional training and to identify those skills, knowledge, and attitudes that most students can reasonably be expected to have mastered before entering the course.

If little or no information is available regarding the students' previous training, the instructor may have to make relatively arbitrary assumptions concerning the entry competencies of students.

Similar to professional competencies and terminal student competencies, entry competencies are best formulated in terms of conditions and performance, as is illustrated by in the example on page A-41.

CROSS-REFERENCE

For additional examples and guidelines on how to identify entry competencies of students, see Problem 10 in Unit B beginning on page B-82.

EXAMPLE

The instructor of the course on pediatric paramedical care decided that experienced pediatric nurses should, on entering the program, have mastered the entry competencies listed at the **bottom** of the following worksheet.

PROFESSIONAL, TERMINAL, AND ENTRY COMPETENCIES

Responsibility No. 1: Takes a complete medical history from parent when appropriate.

CONDITIONS	PERFORMANCE
Professional Competency: When given a variety of pediatric cases in a clinical setting, history forms, and any needed decision guides. . .	. . . practitioners determine when complete medical histories are needed, put patients and parents at ease, take histories, and record data on history forms.
Terminal Student Competency: When given a fellow student who has been primed with a patient scenario in a classroom setting, a history form, and any needed decision guides.	. . . students will put the "parent" at ease, take a complete medical history, and record the data on the history form.
Entry Student Competencies: When given. . . (a) . . . a list of common signs and symptoms. . . (b) . . . a list of organ systems and a randomized list of the different parts within these systems . . . (c) multiple-choice questions related to: — the basic disease process — gestation periods — abortions, etc. . .	Students will . . . . . . give common-sense definitions or explanations of 75% of the terms. . . . match parts to system in which they belong with 80% accuracy. . . . select correct answers in 75% of the cases.

Describe Terminal Student Competencies

1. Describe professional conditions and performance.

2. Plan simulation of professional conditions and performance, taking into consideration:

   a. Entry competencies

   c. Needs for evaluation

b. Resources for Simulation

When considering ways of simulating the professional setting in the classroom, the instructor must take into account the range of resources which are available; that is:

"How much time, money, facilities, and personnel are available to implement the simulation procedures?"

There is no point in planning simulations procedures that will not be feasible to implement within the constraints of the course. As the instructor considers each successively lower level of simulation for inclusion as the terminal student competency, he/she should ask the following types of questions:

TIME
- Is there sufficient time for each student to demonstrate the competency?
- Is there sufficient time to obtain and to prepare materials needed for the simulation (e.g., case materials, sample forms, etc)?

MONEY
- Are there sufficient funds available to purchase any accessories required for the simulation (e.g., samples, slides, mannequins, laboratory equipment, etc)?
- Are there any outside sources of funds that could be tapped (e.g., grants from government or industry, students, etc)?

FACILITIES
- Are existing facilities appropriate for the simulation procedures?
- Is there sufficient space for setting up and carrying out the simulation?
- Are requisite lab services, audiovisual equipment, etc., available?

PERSONNEL
- Are additional staff necessary and available to help organize and administer the simulation procedures?
- Are patients available who both exhibit the requisite characteristics and are willing to cooperate?

Describe Ter-
minal Student
Competencies

1. Describe
   profes-
   sional con-
   ditions and
   perfor-
   mance.

2. Plan simu-
   lation of
   profes-
   sional con-
   ditions and
   perfor-
   mance, tak-
   ing into
   considera-
   tion:

   a. Entry
      compe-
      tencies
   b. Re-
      sources
      for sim-
      ulation

**CROSS-
REFERENCE**

c. Needs for Evaluation

The final consideration in determining the highest level of simulation for a terminal student competency is the feasibility of evaluating that level of competency in the instructional setting.

If an instructor is to be accountable, it is not sufficient to specify **what** the students will learn to do without also specifying **how** that student learning will be assessed. That is, how will the instructor and the students know if the students have successfully achieved the terminal competencies?

Describing student competencies in terms of conditions and performance gives them the appearance of "test items." This is because these competencies should be evaluated at some point during or at the end of the instruction. The question here is whether or not the competency as stated can be incorporated into a formal test for assessing achievement of that competency.

As used here, the term **test** includes all forms of evaluation procedures. It does **not** mean merely paper-and-pencil exams. Rather, it means any kind of formal evaluation, which **may** be a paper-and-pencil test but may also be a practical exam, an oral exam, a project assignment, or a computer-mediated simulation of diagnostic and treatment problems.

Chapter 8 in Unit C provides additional information concerning testing. Specific evaluation techniques are described and compared; and issues such as validity, reliability, and grading are considered.

There are three main kinds of tests to be considered: posttests, pretests, and prerequisite tests. Their relation to the instructional process is depicted in the diagram shown below.

THE RELATIONSHIP BETWEEN FORMAL TESTS AND INSTRUCTION

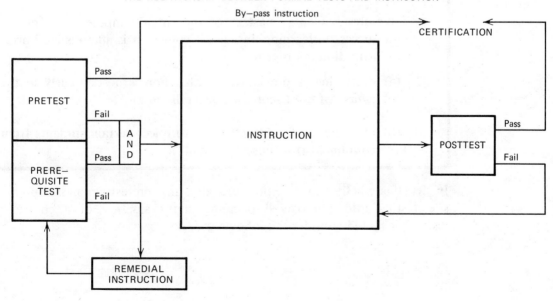

DEFINITION

> **POSTTEST**
>
> — Measures the extent to which students have attained the specified terminal competencies *after* a unit of instruction, in order to
>
> (a) "certify" satisfactory completion of a course or to assign grades, and/or
>
> (b) revise the instructional process on the basis of what students did and did not learn adequately from the instruction.

DEFINITION

> **PRETEST**
>
> — Measures the extent to which students have attained the terminal competencies *before* a unit of instruction, in order to:
>
> (a) select students who need the instruction (low scores),
>
> (b) identify and offer suggestions to those who may bypass instruction (very high scores),
>
> (c) establish tracks of learning for certain groups (for those who score high or low on certain parts of the pretest).
>
> (d) assign individualized or self-paced materials if the course is not group-paced (depending on individual strengths and weaknesses).

DEFINITION

> **PREREQUISITE TEST**
>
> — Measures students' mastery of the entry competencies *required* for successful learning during the course. It is administered prior to instruction in order to:
>
> (a) determine if preparatory instruction is needed early in the course (if most scores are generally low),
>
> (b) offer remedial instruction or to reject certain students from enrollment (for those who "fail").

In deciding whether to incorporate posttesting, pretesting, and/or prerequisite testing into the overall planning and evaluation of a course, the instructor should consider the following:

(a) *Posttests.* Ideally, each terminal student competency should be represented by a formal posttest. The posttest should be based on the conditions and performance specified for that terminal competency. In effect, the terminal competency is a set of specifications for the posttest that will be used to evaluate attainment of that competency. Thus, when determining the highest level of simulation for a terminal student competency, instructors should modify the conditions and performance to conform to a feasible test procedure.

(b) *Pretests.* Ideally, pretesting is done to permit bypassing of instruction as appropriate (to enable students who have already mastered a competency to avoid "reinstruction"). Thus, the pretest should, in theory, be identical to the posttest. In practice, however, pretests may be alternate or shorter versions of the posttest. Pretesting should *not* be done routinely; it can be both onerous and time-consuming. Pretesting should be used only when (1) there are likely to be substantial differences in entry levels, and (2) individualization of instruction is feasible.

(c) *Prerequisite tests.* Ideally, prerequisite testing is done to ensure that students do not enter instruction unless they are adequately prepared and to enable those who lack specific prerequisites to be given appropriate remedial help. In practice, prerequisite testing is functional only if the results can be implemented; for example, by providing general "remedial" coverage where a large number of students prove lacking in specific prerequisites and/or individualized remedial instruction for particular individuals.

Many course designers are reluctant to include formal posttesting in their courses. This reluctance is based, usually, on the assumption that posttests are always characterized by arbitrarily determined fact-recall questions which often fail to deal directly with competencies genuinely relevant to the requirements of professional performance. The hope here is that through systematic course design—with posttests used to assess attainment of terminal student competencies that reflect (are based on and simulate) professional competencies—the instructor can move beyond fact-recall testing to assessments of competencies that are relevant to the future professional needs of the students.

CROSS-REFERENCE

Problem 11 in Unit B deals with the effective use of pretests, posttests, and prerequisite tests. Beginning on page B-88, this section provides several exercises on how to interpret and use the data from these types of tests.

PHASE 2: DESCRIBING STUDENT COMPETENCIES

TASKS	PROCEDURES	PRODUCTS
1. Describe professional conditions and performance.	For each responsibility for which instruction is to be planned, summarize: a. typical **conditions** under which the responsibility is executed in the professional setting, and b. the **performance** of a competent practitioner discharging the responsibility under those conditions.	Descriptions of the **professional competencies** associated with each responsibility to be taught.
2. Plan simulation of the professional conditions and performance.	Determine **feasible** and **assessible** conditions and performance that most closely apploximate the professional conditions and performance. Take into consideration: a. the entry competencies of the students, b. the resources available for simulation, and c. the needs for formal evaluation (i.e., posttests, pretests, and/or prerequistie ts and/or prerequisite tests). If you have difficulty with this step, consult Problems 9, 10, and 11 in Unit B beginning on page B-70. Also, consult Chapter 8 in Unit C for details on specific evaluation techniques and related issues (page C-29).	*Descriptions of **entry** and **terminal student competencies** for each professional competency. Below is shown a suggested format for displaying these competencies.

*Needed in subsequent steps of the course design model.

SUGGESTED FORMAT

(For Describing Student Competencies)

Course Title: _____

PROFESSIONAL, TERMINAL, AND ENTRY COMPETENCIES

Responsibility: _____

CONDITIONS	PERFORMANCE
Professional Competency: When given _____ ...	... practitioners _____.
Terminal Student Competency: When given _____ ...	...students will _____.
Entry Student Competencies: When given: ... (a) ... _____ ... (b) ... _____ ...	Students will ... ... _____. ... ... _____.

WHERE ARE WE? Phase 2 of the course design model is completed when conditions and performances have been specified for each terminal student competency for which instruction is to be planned.

These specifications of the terminal competencies expected of students represent the end points of the instruction, and, as such, the instructional objectives for the course. They are also referred to as **competency-based** objectives, since they are derived from an analysis of the future professional competencies and prior entry competencies of the students.

By now it should be evident that the term **competency** has a special meaning within the context of the course design model.

DEFINITION

COMPETENCY

— **The ability to *perform* certain behaviors when presented with a particular set of conditions.**

— **A specific capability or proficiency defined in terms of "conditions" and "performance."**

Thus far we have been concerned with three types of competencies, as depicted in the diagram below.

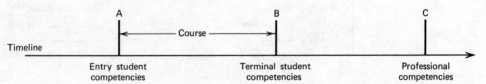

Phase 3 of the course design model is concerned with what takes place between the entry and terminal competencies. The next chapter describes how to plan a sequence of instructional activities for having students progress from point A to point B on the above diagram.

Chapter 3

OVERVIEW OF PHASE 3: PLANNING STUDENT LEARNING

Contents

INTRODUCTION

"As I consider how to teach the course, I fear my choice of classroom activities will be limited to those to which I've been exposed and with which I feel comfortable."

*"Somehow this doesn't seem very systematic. But how **should** I design activities for the desired learning?"*

The instructor has now reached perhaps the most crucial stage in designing his course, for in planning the instruction, his decisions not only will affect whether the desired learning takes place, but also will determine the dynamics of the learning environment; that is, whether information is merely transmitted or students assume significant responsibility for their own learning; whether students merely observe, listen, and ask questions or whether they also demonstrate, explain, and answer questions.

If an instructor wants students to be able to list the major known causes of stroke, they can listen to a lecture and/or read about the causes. But if the terminal student competency is to diagnose and prescribe treatment for high blood pressure, are lectures and readings alone sufficient? Surely students need to practice taking blood pressures, ordering tests, interpreting test results in the context of medical histories, choosing among alternate treatment regimes, etc. What kinds of learning activities are required to enable students to meet this objective, besides lectures and reading?

CHAPTER PURPOSE

The purpose of this chapter is to outline a method for planning student learning and developing a course syllabus.

The major tasks of Phase 3 are:

1. To define intermediate competencies for checking student progress.
2. To design instructional activities to facilitate students' acquisition of the intermediate and terminal competencies.
3. To develop the course syllabus.

At this point in the systematic course design model, the course designer has described the required entry competencies and desired terminal competency for each responsibility in the mastery description for which instruction is to be planned. These two levels of competence also define the boundaries of a "unit of instruction."

DEFINITION

UNIT OF INSTRUCTION

– All instructional activities related to a single responsibility from the mastery description and designed to facilitate student progress from entry level to desired terminal competence.

To ensure that the next task of course design is manageable, regardless of the scope or complexity of the course, the procedures for planning instruction will be discussed in relation to only one unit of instruction, that is, one terminal competency at a time. Later, the instructional activities for the entire set of terminal competencies will be considered collectively for developing the course syllabus.

The tasks for developing a unit of instruction (Tasks 1 and 2 of this chapter) require that:

(a) intermediate competencies be defined to assess student progress at appropriate points between the entry competencies and the terminal competency, and

(b) instructional activities then be designed to enable students to develop each of these competencies.

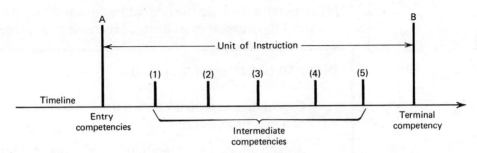

The next section describes how to define intermediate competencies.

Plan Student
Learning

2. Design in-
   structional
   activities.

3. Develop
   course
   syllabus.

1. Define Intermediate Competencies

In deciding how to facilitate student learning from entry to terminal competence, it is useful to identify a number of **intermediate competencies** to be used as checkpoints during the instruction to:

(a) determine whether the desired learning is taking place, and

(b) provide feedback to students concerning their progress.

DEFINITION

INTERMEDIATE COMPETENCIES

— **Capabilities expected of students at various points *before* the end of a unit of instruction.**

— **Specifications of "conditions" and "performance" at levels of simulation *below* that of the terminal competency and *above* that of the entry competencies.**

— **Proficiencies related to specific skill, knowledge, and/or attitude components of a responsibility, or to combinations of these components.**

As with the definition of entry and terminal competencies, intermediate competencies are defined in terms of the conditions under which student progress will be assessed and the desired student performance under these conditions. Keeping in mind that terminal competencies represent the **highest** level of simulation associated with a unit of instruction, and entry competencies represent the lowest levels of simulation, it follows that intermediate competencies represent **intermediate levels of simulation.**

When determining intermediate competencies, as when determining a terminal competency, the instructor must take into consideration:

(a) entry competencies,

(b) available resources for simulation, and

(c) the needs for evaluating performance at one level of simulation before allowing students to practice at the next higher level of simulation.

With the above in mind, the instructor should review the revised mastery description, and for each responsibility decide:

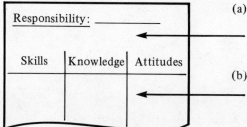

(a) Is it desirable and feasible to assess students' mastery of the **entire** responsibility at one or more levels of simulation **below** that of the terminal competency?

(b) Should students' mastery of any specific **components** skill, knowledge, and/or attitude be confirmed at some point in the instructional process?

Those intermediate competencies closest to the terminal competence will most likely involve lower levels of simulation of the **entire** responsibility, while intermediate competencies close to entry may involve the students' mastery of only isolated **components** of the responsibility, as is illustrated below.

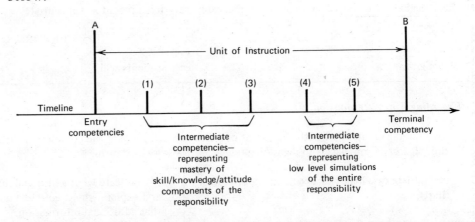

EXAMPLE

On the next page are shown the intermediate competencies defined for the pediatric paramedic's responsibility of "taking a complete medical history from the parent when appropriate." The first two were developed for the entire responsibility, and the remaining seven were developed for isolated skill, knowledge, and attitude components of that responsibility.

To visualize how these intermediate competencies fit into the overall unit of instruction for this responsibility, refer to the Professional, Terminal, and Entry Competencies described on page A-41.

INTERMEDIATE COMPETENCIES

Responsibility No. 1: Takes a complete medical history from parent as appropriate.

CONDITIONS	PERFORMANCE
When given . . .	Students will . . .

(Regarding Entire Responsibility:)	
1. An audiotaped interview with the parent of a sick child; history form; access to decision guides . . .	. . . record the complete medical history on the history form
2. Incomplete case histories; access to decision flow-charts. . . .	. . . indicate what additional information is needed and explain why it could be important to have that additional information.
(Regarding Isolated Components:)	
3. a. List of common chief complaints (e.g., baby has a cold; baby not eating, etc.); plus access to decision flowcharts . . .	a. . . . list a question series to explore each chief complaint, excluding any factors not directly related to the chief complaint.
b. Additional history data about the patient (e.g., 3-month-old white male baby born premature) . . .	b. . . . list additional questions that should be asked in light of the additional information.
4. Directions . . .	. . . reconstruct from memory the standard immunization routine.
5. A list of most important developmental milestones plus other attained skills not considered standard neonatal milestones . . .	. . . indicate which are the important neonatal milestones and give appropriate age for achieving each of these milestones.
6. A list of all persons and pertinent diseases in three generations of a family . . .	. . . construct a medical family tree.
7. Brief descriptions of social history for particular cases . . .	. . . indicate special diagnostic considerations and implications for therapy and patient compliance.
8. A list of general organ systems . . .	. . . list common complaints involving each of these systems.
9. Multiple-choice questions . . .	. . . recognize: – when a complete history is needed – leading and nonleading questions – definitions of gravity, parity, gestation, etc. – importance of birth history, family history, etc.

The conditions and performances that define the intermediate competencies provide, in effect, specifications for **progress tests** to measure student learning **during** the instructional process.

DEFINITION

PROGRESS TESTS

– Any explicit assessment of student performance defined by an intermediate competency can include:

(a) *Brief checktests*–often incorporated with other instructional activities in a given session and providing rapid feedback to both the instructor and student (e.g., after demonstrating the calculation of "relative" and "attributable risk," biostatistics students may be asked to calculate these measures of risk, given a representative problem).

(b) *Teaching observations*–an intrinsic part of almost all instruction involving the direct observation of students (e.g., watching and rating laboratory work, observing classroom participation, or reviewing student answers to programmed material).

(c) *Selftests*–by which students can assess their own progress (perhaps with the aid of another student or reference aids such as a textbook).

Progress testing completes the overall evaluation plan as depicted in the diagram below.

A GENERAL EVALUATION PLAN

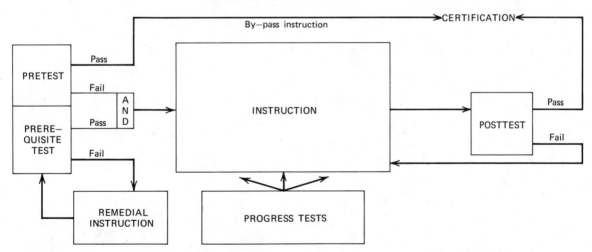

SUMMARY OF RELATION-SHIPS BETWEEN TESTS AND COMPETENCIES

It is helpful to recall that . . .

The following student competencies:		*Provide specifications for the following types of tests:*
ENTRY	⟶	Prerequisite tests
INTERMEDIATE	⟶	Progress tests
TERMINAL	⟶	Posttests (and Pretests)

CROSS-REFERENCE

For additional examples and guidelines for identifying intermediate competencies, see Problem 12 in Unit B (page B-100).

Plan Student
Learning

1. Define in-
   termediate
   compe-
   tencies.

3. Develop
   course
   syllabus.

DEFINITION

2. Design Instructional Activities

Now that the teacher has decided precisely what competencies will be expected of students at various points in the instructional process, the next task is to decide what instructional activities are necessary to enable students to learn these competencies.

INSTRUCTIONAL ACTIVITY

— Any teaching or learning activity designed to serve one or more instructional functions to facilitate student progress through a unit of instruction.

— Generally focused on helping students develop the skills, knowledge, and/or attitudes required for a particular intermediate or terminal competency.

In general, one or more instructional activities will need to be planned to facilitate the learning of each intermediate competency identified for an instructional unit.

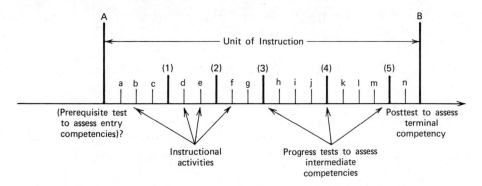

In the above figure, notice that a unit of instruction is composed of a series of events; that is, groups of instructional activities alternating with evaluation activities to assess the competencies being learned.

How does a teacher decide what instructional activities are needed?

Seldom is there only one way to teach any given competency, but usually there are appropriate and inappropriate instructional activities in view of:

(a) where the students are in the learning process, and
(b) the desired student learning to be facilitated by the activity.

It is important then for the course designer to understand that the choice of an instructional activity must be based in part on how that activity will **function** to facilitate student learning, and that certain types of activities are more likely than others to serve a particular **instructional function**.

DEFINITION

INSTRUCTIONAL FUNCTION

— The part or role played by an instructional activity in the context of the instructional unit.

— The way in which an instructional activity facilitates student progress at a specific point in the learning process.

The table on the following two pages describes seven instructional functions. This table should be used as a guide when developing instructional activities for intermediate competencies.

Beginning with the entry competencies and looking toward the first intermediate competency, the instructor should ask him/herself: For what instructional functions must I design activities? That is:

- Do I need **to provide a frame of reference** for this competency?

- Do I need to provide students with a **reason to learn** this competency?

- Do they need an opportunity **to practice** before they can pass satisfactorily a progress test based on this competency?

- Do they need a **demonstration** before they can practice, or will verbal directions suffice?

- Must I provide **feedback** on their performance?

TABLE OF INSTRUCTIONAL FUNCTIONS

INSTRUCTIONAL FUNCTIONS	EXPLANATION OF FUNCTION	EXAMPLES OF APPROPRIATE INSTRUCTIONAL ACTIVITIES
1. Providing a frame of reference.	Setting behaviors to be learned in context; reviewing old material; overviewing new material; providing a transition from old material to new.	— Oral explanation of how the material relates to the students' future professional responsibilities. — Film, videotape or case study setting the stage for a unit of instruction.
2. Providing a reason to learn.	Initiating motivation; facilitating students' readiness to learn; arousing curiosity.	— Group discussion which encourages students to link critical issues with their past or probable future. — Film or slides depicting advantages of learning the material, or the consequences of failing to learn. — Trigger film (open-ended film) which allows students to speculate about cause-effect, probable outcomes, etc.
3. Shaping student attitudes.	Reinforcing students' approximation of the desired attitude or value; allowing students to express behaviors consonant with the attitude or quality; overcoming negative attitudes.	— Instructor models or exhibits the desired qualities, attitudes or behaviors throughout instruction. — Provide real or simulated experiences via T-groups, on-the-job visits, discussions, role reversals, simulation games.
4. Transmitting information.	Providing students with basic knowledge such as technical vocabulary, criteria for decisions, or underlying facts, concepts and theories; providing procedural steps for performing a specific task; increasing student awareness.	— Handouts, programmed materials, texts, etc. — Supplementing learning with decision flow charts, procedural guidelines, worksheets.
5. Demonstrating behaviors to be learned.	Modeling behaviors to be learned; reproducing and displaying the product of a process.	— **Live** classroom demonstrations by instructor, students or guests using real or simulated stimuli. — **Canned** demonstrations on audiotape, film, videotape or slides.

(table continued)

INSTRUCTIONAL FUNCTIONS	EXPLANATION OF FUNCTION	EXAMPLES OF APPROPRIATE INSTRUCTIONAL ACTIVITIES

6. Allowing students to practice behaviors	Allowing students to perform at various levels of simulation; may involve prompting or guiding student performance.	– Have students:
		  – read case studies and practice solving problems,
		  – play roles or participate in simulation games,
		  – perform laboratory exercises and write up project reports,
		  – work through programmed exercises,
		  – participate in on-the-job assignments.

7. Providing feedback on student progress	Responding to students by commenting on the quality of their performance; transmitting written, verbal, or nonverbal assessment of student behavior.	– Learner is placed in representative problem situation requiring competencies which he is expected to have learned. – Instructor administers observation tests, practical exams, quizzes, etc., with feedback provided. – Giving feedback during any observation of student practice (including on-the-spot coaching).

PARTIAL EXAMPLE

Intermediate Competency

When given the types of vaccines, students will describe the contraindications and ways to deal with each.

Instructional Activities

– Describe outcomes of immunized patients for whom contraindications were *not* considered (*to provide a frame of reference **and** a reason to learn*).

– Have students read a handout describing contraindications and ways to deal with them for each type of vaccine (*to transmit information*).

– In class, briefly discuss each vaccine, intermittently asking students to recall specific details from the handout as in a programmed lecture (*for allowing students to practice and providing feedback*).

GUIDELINES FOR DESIGNING INSTRUCTIONAL ACTIVITIES

1. *Getting Started.* Review the entire range of intermediate competencies defined for a unit of instruction and decide which competencies should be taught first. Put the other competencies in an approximate order for instruction. This need not represent the final instructional sequence within the unit, since one tends to revise and reorder activities frequently as one comes closer to the final syllabus.

2. *Using the Mastery Description.* The analyzed responsibility in the revised mastery description is an essential reference when designing instructional activities. The skill, knowledge, and attitude components of this analysis provide the instructor with the substantive information needed to enable students to attain the terminal competency. All essential components of the responsibility should be included in some instructional activity at some point in the associated unit of instruction.

3. *Assessment.* Include evaluation activities when needed to:

   (a) assess entry competence (pretest and prerequisite test),
   (b) provide feedback on student progress (progress tests),
   (c) assess terminal competence (posttest)

4. *Introductions.* Early in the unit of instruction, include activities to:

   (a) provide a frame of reference for the entire responsibility, and
   (b) provide a reason to learn the terminal competency.

5. *Maximizing Use of Class Time.* When possible, plan activities that transmit information on an individualized basis (perhaps outside reading). Emphasize other teaching functions for activities within the instructional setting, especially if the instruction is generally group-paced.

6. *Demonstration and Practice.* When appropriate, demonstrate new skills before requiring students to practice them. Demonstrations are a good way to "shape student attitudes," since the desired qualities and behaviors can be modeled during a demonstration. Be sure to allow students to practice skills before the final evaluation of these skills.

EXAMPLE

The following pages show the instructional activities developed for an entire unit of instruction for the course on pediatric paramedical care. Two or more instructional activities have been planned to:

   (a) introduce the unit as a whole,
   (b) facilitate student learning of each intermediate competency, and
   (c) facilitate progress toward the terminal competency.

INSTRUCTIONAL UNIT

<u>Responsibility No. 1:</u> Takes a complete medical history from parent when appropriate.

COMPETENCIES	INSTRUCTIONAL ACTIVITIES
(Introduction to the unit of instruction)	– Have students examine a completed history form and try to determine what the advantages of using such a form might be. – Show videotaped demonstration of complete history-taking interview, using the same case material as shown on the completed history form examined above.
*IC # 5 Given list of *milestones*, students will identify the most important and give ages for achievement.	– Have students read handout on growth and development. – Orally review the most important milestones to be memorized for convenience. – Explain the Denver Developmental Aptitude Test. – Have students list appropriate milestones for a list of given ages.
IC # 4 Students will reconstruct from memory the standard *immunization routine.*	– Have students read a handout that includes presentation and explanation of standard immunization routine. – Orally review immunization schedule, pointing out convenience of committing it to memory. – Have students practice recalling the immunization routine.
IC # 6 Given three generations of a case family, students will construct a *medical family tree.*	– Show family tree on completed history form and explain symbols; ask students about potential importance of family tree. – Using guidesheet, demonstrate construction of family tree for student volunteer. – Have students practice constructing trees and comparing results on blackboard.
IC # 7 Given cases of *social histories*, students will indicate special diagnostic considerations and implications for therapy and patient compliance.	– Have students read handout describing how to take a social history, and implications of particular types of responses. – Have students discuss possible diagnostic considerations and implications of particular social case histories.

Handwritten margin notes: Providing a reason to learn · Providing a frame of reference · Transmitting information · allowing student practice · Providing feedback · allowing student practice

*"IC # 5" means "the fifth intermediate competency listed on page A-54. Notice that the instructor has revised the order of the competencies for teaching purposes.

(Instructional Unit, continued)

COMPETENCIES	INSTRUCTIONAL ACTIVITIES
IC # 9 Given multiple-choice items, students will recognize: – when a complete history is necessary, – leading and nonleading questions, – definitions of gravity, parity, gestation, etc. – importance of birth history, family history, etc.	– In a class discussion, have students figure out what types of visits do and do not require a complete history. – In discussion, have students practice recognizing differences between leading and nonleading questions and explain why it matters. – Have students read handout giving these definitions, and review them as they come up during class. – Have students read handout describing questions to ask in taking each part of the history, and implications of usual types of answers to questions. – In class discussion, have students determine importance of each type of question and why it needs to be asked.
IC # 8 Given list of general *organ systems*, students will list common complaints involved in each system.	– Have students read handout describing common complaints involving each organ system as well as the specific questions to be asked to elicit problems related to the systems. – Review handout stressing importance of organ systems review in subsequent visits.
IC # 3 Given *common chief complaints*, students will list question series to explore complaint, and then, upon being given additional history data, will list additional questions that should be asked in light of the new data.	– Have students study a set of decision flow charts giving what questions to ask in exploring details of common chief complaints. – Demonstrate use of decision flow charts. – Have students practice exploring chief complaints using the flow charts (in pairs, one student primed with patient scenario). – Have students practice using the charts to list appropriate question series for particular chief complaints plus some additional case history data.
IC # 1 Given audiotaped interview with parent of sick child, students will record history data on a history form.	– Have students read handout listing specific questions to be asked in taking a history, how to ask and rephrase these questions, and how to record the responses onto the history form. – Demonstrate process of recording interview responses on history form. – Have students practice recording histories from audiotaped patient interviews.

Handwritten annotations: Providing a frame of reference; Providing a reason to learn; Reviewing learning; Demonstrate Procedures; Allowing Practice; Modeling behaviors

COMPETENCIES	INSTRUCTIONAL ACTIVITIES
IC # 2 Given incomplete case histories, students will indicate what additional information is needed and explain why it is important.	— After limited practice recording case histories as above, have students analyze incomplete case history forms, and determine what additional questions should have been asked. — In small groups, have students discuss the incomplete histories analyzed independently above.
Terminal Competency Given a classmate primed with a patient scenario, students will take a complete medical history on the history form.	— In groups of three and then in pairs, have students practice taking histories on classmates primed with scenarios. Have interviews tape-recorded and on replay, have other students give feedback before instructor comments. — Have students practice taking complete histories from actual patients under supervision of an intern or resident.

Providing feedback

allowing practice at high level of simulation

*"Five weeks of human anatomy and all I've done is **memorize** every bone in the body! Is this course just an academic exercise in memorization?"*

A word of caution . . . There is sometimes a tendency to teach all the knowledge components early in the unit on the assumption that students must be saturated with facts, information, theory, and concepts **before** they are able to practice applications. The result is generally a passive learning environment with emphasis on the instructor "transmitting" and students "memorizing." Students rapidly lose interest, unable to grasp the relevance of the material, anxious to demonstrate new skills and capabilities.

To avoid this tendency whenever possible, distribute activities that transmit knowledge throughout the unit of instruction, and allow students to practice applications and obtain feedback on their performance early as well as later in the learning process.

SELECTING METHODS AND MEDIA

Although any teacher is generally more comfortable when using instructional methods and media that are familiar, the main criterion for designing instructional activities should not be "comfort" or "expertise." Rather, instructional activities should be designed by selecting methods and media that are **appropriate** for the desired instructional **function**; that is, methods and media to facilitate the desired outcome at a specific point in the learning process. It is the responsibility of the instructor to increase his/her repertoir of teaching skills to accomodate appropriate instructional activities.

EXAMPLE

To teach people how to administer cardiopulmonary resuscitation (CPR), various instructional packages are available including programmed texts, slide-tape shows, movies, overhead transparencies, and mannequin. The mannequin is designed to simulate human characteristics and responses.

If the instructional function is merely to "provide a frame of reference," "provide a reason to learn," or "transmit information" about CPR, any of the above suggested activities (using programmed texts, showing slide-tape shows, etc.) might be appropriate for instruction.

However, if students already understand the procedures of CPR and are motivated to apply their learning, and if the desired instructional functions are to "demonstrate" and "allow student practice," utilizing the mannequin for demonstration and practice will not only facilitate students acquiring the desired skills, but may also help "shape student attitudes" by overcoming underlying fears and reservations (such as human oral or nasal contact, danger of breaking or cracking ribs, uncertainty of proper rhythm for compressions, etc).

CROSS-REFERENCES

For additional examples and guidelines on how to design instructional activities for a unit of instruction, see Problem 13 of Unit B, page B-113.

Chapter 9 in Unit C, beginning on page C-54, describes a variety of specific methods and media that are useful when designing instructional activities; and Problem 14 in Unit B, page B-130, provides additional guidelines for the selection of appropriate methods and media.

Planning Stu-
dent Learning

1. Define
   intermedi-
   ate compe-
   tencies
2. Design
   instruc-
   tional
   activities.

3. Develop Course Syllabus

Once the teacher has planned each unit of instruction by specifying the instructional activities necessary for each intermediate competency, all the units must be considered collectively to finalize the order in which the activities will be implemented during instruction.

This final sequence of instructional activities is described by a course syllabus. Although the process of developing the syllabus from the individual units of instruction may be somewhat mechanical (i.e., fitting "x" number of activities into "y" number of hours for instruction), there are several important guidelines to consider when finalizing the course design via its syllabus:

(a) Are there instructional activities **not** associated with specific competencies but required to ensure the effectiveness of the course and of the units comprising it? For example:

- Providing frames of reference and reasons for learning at the start of the course.
- Providing evaluation activities that integrate previously learned components and provide for better retention.
- Providing periodic review and preview activities to ensure that students have a clear picture at all times of where they are in the instruction.

(b) How should one **sequence** the instructional units (and activities within them) to facilitate progressive development of the terminal competencies for the course?

- Is there a "logical" sequence for the units and activities?
- Are course segments that are prerequisite to others introduced prior to those others?
- Are there any units or activities that might facilitate the total learning experience by occurring early?
- Are there segments within different units which may be confusing if taught separately, and should thus be taught at the same time?
- Might students be motivated by a **demonstration** of certain skills at a high level of simulation before they **practice** those skills at lower levels of simulation?
- Should evaluation activities from several different units be **combined** and administered simultaneously in a formal exam?

(c) What instructional activities could be done **outside** the instructional setting, and which should take place in class?

- Which activities involve reading, doing research, working on individual or group projects, etc.?

- Can any of the activities which were designed primarily to "transmit information" be converted to outside assignments to free more in-class time for other instructional functions?

EXAMPLE

The partial course syllabus on the following pages is based on the instructional unit for the pediatric paramedical course as outlined on pages A-62 to A-64.

CROSS-REFERENCES

See Problem 15 in Unit B (page B-137) for additional examples and guidelines concerning the development of a syllabus. See Problem 16 (page B-142) for guidelines on how to design the first class session.

PARTIAL SYLLABUS

Course Title: Pediatric Paramedical Care
Unit Title: Taking Medical Histories

Lashley University
1974-1975

Date	Instructional Activities	Assignment for Next Session
Session 1 Sept. 24 (2 hr)	**– Introduction to Course.** Student introductions, review of syllabus, administrative details, etc. **– Instructor-led Discussion.** Major features, role, and importance of history form (centered on blank copy of form plus filled-in model form). **– Videotaped Demonstration.** Complete parent interview (same as model case). **– Instructor-led Discussion.** Of videotape, appropriate occasions for complete history, getting started (putting patient at ease, etc.)	Reading **Handout A** (on growth and development, including Denver Developmental Aptitude Test).
Session 2 Sept. 26 (2 hr)	**– Mini-lecture.** Review Handout A pointing out aspects to commit to memory for convenience; explain DDAT; walk students through Handout B explaining important aspects. **– Instructor-led discussion.** Interview techniques (direct questioning; leading vs. non-leading questions, etc.) **– Exercise.** Have students practice recalling milestones and immunization routine. Discuss results immediately in class.	Study **Handout B** (a listing of questions to be asked for each category of history form, how to ask and rephrase these questions, important definitions, how to record responses, and explanations of common or noteworthy answers).
Lab A Sept. 28 (3 hr)	**– Instructor-led Discussion.** On Handout B with emphasis on Family and Social History including implications for treatment. **– Live Demonstration.** Construction of a family tree using guidelines in Handout B. **– Exercise.** Students practice constructing family trees; receive feedback. **– Exercise.** Students practice recording answers to family and social history questions from taped patient interviews; implications of each case discussed as feedback is given after each case.	Read **Handout C** (describing common complaints involving each organ system). Review "Systems Review" section of Handout B. Study sample **Decision Flowchart** (giving questions to ask in exploring common chief complaints related to respiratory system)*

*Additional Decision Flowcharts will be provided later in course as part of each major organ system.

(Partial Syllabus, continued)

Date	Instructional Activities	Assignment for Next Session
Session 3 Oct. 1 (2 hr)	— **Mini-lecture.** Review Handout C stressing importance of systems review at all visits. — **Live Demonstration.** Use of Decision Flowchart to explore hypothetical chief complaints and to record results on history form. — **Practice Interviews.** In pairs, using sample Flowchart and patient scenarios, students explore chief complaints and record responses on form (instructor feedback).	**Exercise-To-Be-Handed-in.** Students list series of questions to explore specified chief complaints with additional complications (may use flowchart). Review parts of Handout B regarding recording data onto history forms.
Session 4 Oct. 3 (2 hr)	— **Live Demonstration.** Recording entire interview on history form. — **Exercise.** Students record complete medical histories from audiotaped patient interviews. Class feedback and discussion.	Review all handouts to prepare for Lab B.
Lab B Oct. 5 (3 hr)	— **Practice Interviews.** In groups of three, students take complete histories from classmates primed with scenarios. Record interviews on audiotape; on replay, feedback from classmates and instructor.	Analyze incomplete case history forms and determine what additional questions should have been asked.
Session 5 Oct. 8 (2 hr)	— **Small Group Discussion.** In groups of four, students discuss assigned incomplete histories, focusing on how missing information could be important. — **Instructor-led Discussion.** Results of small group discussion compared with critical feedback. — **Practice Interviews.** In pairs and using patient scenarios, students take complete medical histories on history form.	Prepare for Lab C and for practical and written exams.
Lab C (any time during week)	— **Practice Interviews—Real Patients.** Assign each student to a pediatric resident. At mutual convenience during week, student obtains complete medical histories from parents of actual patients under care of resident. Feedback from resident.	Prepare for practical and written exams.
Session 6 Oct. 12 (3 hr)	— **Practical Exam.** Students take complete medical histories from primed classmates (Terminal Competency for unit) — **Written Exam.** Items sampling the intermediate competencies for unit.	

GUIDANCE SYSTEM

PHASE 3: PLANNING STUDENT LEARNING

TASKS	PROCEDURES	PRODUCTS
1. Define intermediate competencies.	For each unit of instruction, specify the **conditions** and **performance** of intermediate levels of simulation for assessing student progress and providing feedback. That is, for each responsibility, determine: a. at what intermediate levels of simulation it is desirable and feasible to check student's mastery of the **entire responsibility**, and b. which skill, knowledge, and/or attitude **components** should be mastered before higher levels of simulation are attempted. For additional guidelines, see page B-100 (Problem 12 in Unit B).	Descriptions of the intermediate competencies for each terminal competency. That is, statements of the conditions and performance for intermediate levels of simulation **above** that of entry and **below** that of the terminal competency. See below for suggested format.
2. Design instructional activities.	a. For each unit of instruction, put intermediate competencies in an approximate sequence for instruction. b. For each intermediate competency, determine what instructional **functions** are needed to facilitate student progress from entry to termination. c. Plan activities to serve appropriate instructional functions, making sure all relevant skill, knowledge, and attitudes are covered. d. If needed, review methods and media in Chapter 9 (page C-54) and guidelines for Problems 13 and 14 in Unit B (pages B-113 and B-130).	Descriptions of instructional activities for each intermediate (and terminal) competency. Should be organized into "units of instruction." See following page for suggested format.
3. Develop course syllabus.	a. Determine final sequence for units of instruction and activities within units. b. Plan activities for continuity between units. c. Identify "assignments" to be done outside the instructional setting. d. Combine and structure in-class and out-of-class activities into the time-frame allotted for the course. e. See page B-141 for additional guidelines.	Course syllabus The following page shows a suggested format for the course syllabus.

SUGGESTED FORMATS

Course Title: _____

INTERMEDIATE COMPETENCIES

Responsibility No.: _____

CONDITIONS	PERFORMANCE
When given . . .	Students will . . .
(Regarding Entire Responsibility:)	
1. . . . _____ . . .	. . . _____ .
2. . . . _____ . . .	. . . _____ .
(Regarding Isolated Components:)	
3. . . . _____ . . .	. . . _____ .
4. . . . _____ . . .	. . . _____ .
5. . . . _____ . . .	. . . _____ .
6. . . . _____ . . .	. . . _____ .

Course Title: _____

INSTRUCTIONAL UNIT

Responsibility No.: _____

COMPETENCIES	INSTRUCTIONAL ACTIVITIES
(Introduction to unit)	_____ _____
IC # -	_____ _____
IC # -	_____ _____
Terminal	_____ _____

SYLLABUS

Course Title: Institution:
Unit Title: Dates:

Date or Session	Instructional Activities	Assignments (Next Session)

WHERE ARE WE? The third (and last) phase of the course design model is completed with the development of the syllabus. The diagram below summarizes the major products associated with the entire course design model.

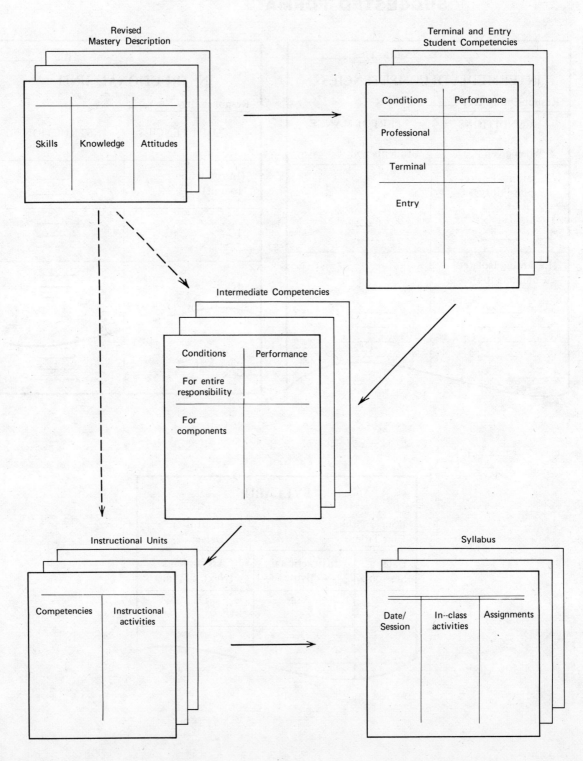

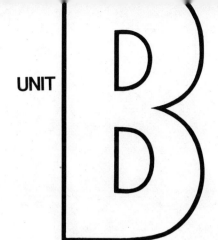

Implementation Problems

Unit B

IMPLEMENTATION PROBLEMS

INTRODUCTION Unit B is intended primarily for those who are actually trying to implement the course design model described in Unit A. The three chapters in Unit B (one for each phase of the model described in Unit A) are organized around specific **problems** that instructors often encounter when trying to apply the course design model to their own instructional situations.

For each problem identified, an effort has been made to provide materials that demonstrate both the nature of the problem and, at least, one way of solving the problem. There are, of course, alternate approaches that could be taken toward the solution of any of these implementation problems, and thus the specific approaches described here in Unit B do not necessarily preclude others.

TYPES OF MATERIALS Each section of Unit B defines a particular implementation problem and includes one or more illustrations of approaches to solving the problem in question. These illustrations may involve any of the following:

- *Mini-Cases*—in which a brief description of an instructional situation containing an implementation problem is followed by one or more questions directed at possible approaches to the problem. Feedback is provided, but readers are encouraged to take a few minutes to answer each question before reading further to how the authors handled the problem.

- *Model Advocate Dialogues*—in which the instructor, who has encountered a particular implementation problem, converses with someone who advocates (or argues for) the use of the course design model. These case studies illustrate the kind of thinking that instructors might find helpful when applying the model to their own situations.

- *Extended Cases*—in which one example is carried through several stages in the model to demonstrate how portions of a course evolve. Usually these extended examples are interspersed with questions to provide opportunities for readers to think through their own ideas for solving specific problems arising in the design process.

- *Feedback Exercises*—which provide structured opportunities for the reader to practice specific skills required for successful application of the model.

In addition to the illustrations, each section begins with an

- *Introduction*—which explains the nature of the problem(s) to be dealt with in the section, and a

- *Directory*—which spells out which illustrations deal with which types of problem on what pages.

Finally, every section concludes with

- *Problem-Solving Guidelines*—which are summaries of the procedures suggested for handling each of the specifically identified and illustrated implementation problems.

HOW TO USE UNIT B

The materials in Unit B may be used in a variety of ways, depending on your needs and learning style. For example, you may find it preferable to:

(a) read the guidelines at the end of a section before looking at any of the illustrations in that section,

(b) work through only those illustrations that seem related to a specific problem you are having in designing a course of your own, and/or

(c) use the illustrations simply as additional examples of various steps in the course design model.

Chapter 4

IMPLEMENTATION PROBLEMS RELATED TO PHASE 1: DESCRIBING PROFESSIONAL PERFORMANCE

SUMMARY OF PHASE 1 OF THE COURSE DESIGN MODEL:

TASK 1
DESCRIBE OPTIMAL PROFESSIONAL PERFORMANCE
1. Identify future professional roles
2. List professional responsibilities
3. Analyze skill/knowledge/attitude components

TASK 2
ANALYZE ACTUAL PROFESSIONAL PERFORMANCE
1. Select and implement method of performance analysis
2. Identify performance discrepancies

TASK 3
REVISE INITIAL DESCRIPTION OF PERFORMANCE
1. Analyze causes of performance discrepancies
2. Modify initial mastery description

IMPLEMENTATION PROBLEMS THAT MAY ARISE: | See Page:

1. What if future roles are widely divergent or unknown? — B-6

2. How does one determine professional responsibilities? — B-12

3. What if it is difficult to determine professional responsibilities? — B-16

4. How does one analyze components of a responsibility? — B-26

5. What if it is difficult to analyze components of a responsibility? — B-39

6. Why choose one method of performance analysis over another? — B-51

7. What if the future role does not currently exist? — B-56

8. How does one conduct a performance analysis and revise the initial mastery description? — B-62

PROBLEM 1

What If Future Professional Roles Are Widely Divergent Or Unknown?

INTRODUCTION

Sometimes it is difficult to identify the future professional roles of students. This may happen because:

(a) the course will include students who will have many different careers, and/or

(b) the course has never been taught before and it has not yet been decided exactly who will enroll.

The materials in this section have been designed to help you learn how to identify roles in these types of situations.

DIRECTORY

TYPE OF PROBLEM	RELATED ILLUSTRATION	SEE PAGE
Multiple student roles	1-A: A Model Advocate Dialogue: Tropical Medicine	B-7
Student population unknown	1-B: A Mini-Case: Hospital Quality Control System	B-9
Summary	Guidelines for Solving Problem 1	B-11

ILLUSTRATION 1-A

A MODEL ADVOCATE DIALOGUE: TROPICAL MEDICINE

Instructor: It would be easy enough to identify future professional roles if most of your students were going to do the same kinds of things. But students who take Tropical Medicine 101 will be doing completely different things. There's no telling when or how they will use what they learn in this course.

Model Advocate: Don't you have **any** idea of what happens to your graduates? Where do they go? What do they do?

Instructor: Oh sure, I have some idea; but not specifically. There are so many possibilities open to them.

Model Advocate: Okay, just give me one example. What is one thing that a student might do?

Instructor: Well, some of them will be directing public health programs of various kinds, but all over the world, not always in the tropics. And their programs will differ widely.

Model Advocate: Could you estimate about how many, in percentage, will end up directing programs, no matter where?

Instructor: Hmmm, well, I suppose about 35% will direct programs in tropical countries; another 15% in nontropical countries—and these may never hear of a tropical disease again. But that may not be true either, because the same individual might move from nontropical to tropical, or vice versa. Besides, some will be conducting research on tropical diseases, and others may simply practice general medicine in America or elsewhere . . . and . . .

Model Advocate: Slow down now, let's back up and see how many students we are talking about. We've already accounted for roughly half of the students. How many go into research or private practice?

Instructor: Well, I guess another 25% will go into research, and let's say 10% will never use the material.

Model Advocate: And what about the last 15%?

Instructor: Oh, they'll probably teach in various schools of medicine or public health, like me.

Model Advocate: I'd say we are ready to summarize the future roles of your students.

(Illustration 1-A, continued)

SUMMARY

FUTURE PROFESSIONAL ROLES

Directors of public health programs in tropics	35%
Directors of health programs in other countries	15%
Research scientists investigating public health problems related to tropical diseases	25%
Teachers in schools of medicine or public health	15%
Physicians in private practice	10%
	100%

ILLUSTRATION 1-B

A MINI-CASE: HOSPITAL QUALITY CONTROL SYSTEM

INSTRUCTIONAL SITUATION

A large city hospital has decided to institute a new quality control record-keeping system. The hospital has asked Dr. Howard, an expert in the new system, to teach a course to train appropriate hospital personnel in the new system. But Dr. Howard does not know, nor has the hospital decided, exactly who will attend the course.

QUESTION 1

Does Dr. Howard need to know who will be taking his course in order to design it? Why do you think so?

FEEDBACK

Without knowing at least what category of personnel will be involved, Dr. Howard has no way of determining the future responsibilities of his students and thus of developing relevant objectives for his course. However, you may think that Dr. Howard merely needs to present an overview of the new system and that competency-based instructional objectives are not necessary. If the course were only for orientation purposes, then we might agree; but if the hospital expects personnel who participate in the course to "do" something afterward that they were not doing beforehand, then these personnel and their future responsibilities must be identified before the course is designed. Thus Dr. Howard must have some idea of who will be taking the course and why, or else he cannot decide whether to develop an orientation course, a course focusing on the development of specific competencies, or some combination of these.

QUESTION 2

How could Dr. Howard determine what specific hospital roles will or should be represented at his course?

FEEDBACK

Dr. Howard needs to have the hospital administration clarify why they want this course taught. What do they expect course participants to do with what they learn? Will they be expected to plan the implementation of the new system for the whole hospital, or simply to change the way they, as individuals, are keeping records at the present time?

(Illustration 1-B, continued)

DR. HOWARD'S SOLUTION

Dr. Howard came up with the following solution to his problem: a matrix within which to enter the hospital administration's answers to his questions. This enabled him to identify the course participants and their needs.

Hospital Personnel	May Attend	Must Attend	Won't Attend	Know About	Know How
Nursing Supervisors					
Ward Clerks					
Filing Clerks					
Director of Billing					
Etc.					

GUIDELINES FOR SOLVING PROBLEM 1

PROBLEM 1   What if future professional roles are widely divergent or unknown?

GUIDELINES

1. If your students are likely to assume a variety of different roles in the future, list as many different types of roles as you can, and estimate the percentage of total students for each role you identify. Asking yourself the following questions might help identify these roles:

   • What kinds of things will my students be doing in the future?

   • What is **one** thing a student might do in the future?

   • What are previous students doing now?

2. If the course has never been taught before and you do not yet know who will enroll, try to determine who **ought** to enroll by asking yourself:

   • Why is the course being taught?

   • What need(s) will be met by this course?

   • Why would someone want to take this course?

3. If appropriate, develop a matrix describing potential course participants, such as that shown for Illustration 1-B above.

PROBLEM 2

How Does One Determine Professional Responsibilities?

INTRODUCTION Sometimes the responsibilities of a professional role are evident to the instructor and thus easy to formulate, but often this is **not** the case. For example:

(a) An instructor may be an expert in the subject area of the course but not in the application of that subject matter within the designated professional context; or

(b) An instructor may be teaching health professionals to teach someone else something about the subject area of one's own expertise (e.g., teaching teachers of nutrition).

The materials in this section have been designed to provide:

(a) a **general procedure** for developing a list of professional responsibilities, and

(b) illustrations of the application of this procedure to the above types of situations.

DIRECTORY

TYPE OF PROBLEM	RELATED ILLUSTRATION	SEE PAGE
The basic procedure	2-A. A Mini-Case: Utilization of Community Resources	B-13
Teaching the teacher	2-B. A Mini-Case: Practical Nutrition	B-14
Summary	Guidelines for Solving Problem 2	B-15

ILLUSTRATION 2-A

A MINI-CASE: UTILIZATION OF COMMUNITY RESOURCES

INSTRUCTIONAL SITUATION

> Dr. Garcia wants to teach a course to medical students on the utilization of community resources. He believes that physicians often fail to refer patients to these sources of assistance in the community because they are not aware of the agencies available or what services are provided by these agencies.
>
> The future professional roles of Dr. Garcia's students are practicing physicians in different medical specialties.

QUESTION

What are the professional responsibilities of Dr. Garcia's students regarding the utilization of community resources?

In answering this question, try to visualize a physician practicing some medical specialty and determine the kinds of things such a practitioner does or should do to effectively utilize service agencies and other community sources of assistance for his/her patients.

FEEDBACK

Below is the list of professional responsibilities actually developed by Dr. Garcia:

The practicing physician (in any speciality) . . .

A. *With respect to Community Agencies and Sources of Assistance*

1. Identifies sources of assistance.
2. Maintains records relative to each source regarding
   − criteria of eligibility for various services
   − routes of access to services
   − patient experiences with source or agency.
3. Contacts agency on behalf of patient when referring, to provide appropriate information about the patient.

B. *With respect to Patients*

1. Determines patient's need for community resources.
2. Decides on optimal management strategy including priorities and alternatives.
3. Identifies impediments to patient's utilization of the resources such as expenses involved, attitudes toward resources, etc.
4. Directs patient to sources of help with careful instructions about the form of assistance that can be expected from each source.
5. Encourages continuing communication from patient.

ILLUSTRATION 2-B

A MINI-CASE: PRACTICAL NUTRITION

INSTRUCTIONAL SITUATION

> The health department of an urban community has decided to use volunteers to train indigent mothers in general health care for their families. The volunteers will work with mothers from the ghetto areas in existing but poorly equipped community health centers. The Commissioner of Health has asked Dr. John Myers to teach a short course on nutrition for these volunteers. (Other experts will be invited to talk about general hygiene, drugs, etc.)

QUESTION

What are the **professional responsibilities** of these volunteer health workers in relation to this short course on nutrition?

FEEDBACK

This case represents a reasonably common instructional situation in which the real target of the training is several steps removed from the instructor; that is, **Dr. Myers** must teach the **volunteer** to teach the **mother** to do something for her **family** regarding nutrition. It is important that the professional responsibilities reflect this relationship. That is, the specific responsibilities of Dr. Myer's students must involve teaching the mothers something about nutrition which they can apply to their families' needs. Some examples of how such responsibilities might be phrased are:

The Volunteer Health Worker . . .

1. Helps mothers plan menus that are not only nutritionally balanced but also tasty and inexpensive.
2. Teaches mothers to purchase nutritious foods on a limited budget.
3. Teaches mothers to store and prepare food so as to preserve its nutritional value.
4. Teaches mothers to recognize signs of malnutrition.
5. Teaches mothers where and how to obtain free professional help with nutritional problems.

GUIDELINES FOR SOLVING PROBLEM 2

PROBLEM 2   How does one proceed in developing a list of professional responsibilities for a specific course?

GUIDELINES   To determine the professional responsibilities for a given role regarding a particular subject area:

1. Try to visualize a competent practitioner in the professional role you have identified, and ask yourself:

   ● What are the major **duties** of this practitioner in relation to the subject matter of this course?

   ● What will this practitioner be **doing** when he/she is using the subject matter of this course?

2. Write down everything that occurs to you as you think about this practitioner performing in his/her role, and then revise and organize your initial listing until you are satisfied that everything has been included.

3. If you have difficulty applying the above guidelines to your particular instructional situation, refer to the materials for Problem 3 which begins on the next page.

PROBLEM 3

What If It Is Difficult To Determine Professional Responsibilities?

INTRODUCTION Sometimes one cannot simply visualize a competent practitioner in action to determine the professional responsibilities for a particular course. This may happen because:

(a) the subject area is a well-defined, traditional part of some "core curriculum,"
(b) more than one different professional role or setting is involved, and/or
(c) the course is an introduction to or survey of a subject area.

The materials in this section have been designed to help you learn how to determine professional responsibilities in situations like these, and when it may **not** be appropriate to use the course design model proposed in this book.

TYPE OF PROBLEM	RELATED ILLUSTRATION	SEE PAGE
Traditional "core curriculum" course	3-A. A Model Advocate Dialogue: Biostatistics	B-17
Multiple roles or settings	3-B. A Mini-Case: Drug Abuse Problems	B-19
Introductory or survey course	3-C. A Mini-Case: Psychology	B-21
Combination of the above factors	3-D A Mini-Case: Physiology	B-23
Summary	Guidelines for Solving Problem 3	B-25

ILLUSTRATION 3-A

A MODEL ADVOCATE DIALOGUE: BIOSTATISTICS

Instructor:	Biostatistics is different! It's just not possible to say how or when dentists will use biostatistics in their future professional roles. They just need to be exposed to it!
Model Advocate:	Why do they need to be exposed to it?
Instructor:	Just because! All good dentists should know certain things about biostatistics. It's simply part of a good background in science.
Model Advocate:	But why? Where would it show up in his practice if a dentist missed out on biostatistics? How would it affect his competence?
Instructor:	(pause) Well, for one thing, he wouldn't be able to draw the proper implications from research reports and journal articles, and his practice would soon become old-fashioned and out-of-date. A good dentist must keep up with the professional literature!
Model Advocate:	Excellent! You've just identified a couple of important professional responsibilities related to this subject matter. That is:

    1. Draws proper implications from research reports and journal articles.
    2. Adopts new dental procedures when supported by adequate research.

Now, are there any others?

Instructor:	Well, if he ever wanted to do a study on his own—to collect and analyze data to test some hypothesis that's bugging him—then he would need his biostatistics!
Model Advocate:	Good! That's a third responsibility for our list:

    3. Collects and analyzes data to test hypotheses.

Now, is there anything else a dentist does that might require some biostatistics?

Instructor:	No, I don't think so . . . but this third responsibility is really more than one responsibility—he's got to design the study, collect data, analyze it and so on. Each of these is a major responsibility by itself!
Model Advocate:	Okay, then write down everything that seems appropriate.

(Illustration 3-A, continued)

SUMMARY

After the instructor listed the responsibilities involved in testing a hypothesis, he realized that his first two responsibilities also needed some revision and expansion. Soon he realized that biostatistics was probably most useful to a dentist when he was actually reading a report on some research study or when he was in the process of testing some hypothesis. His final list of professional responsibilities then became as follows:

A dentist . . .

A. *When reading reports of research studies:*

1. Identifies the purpose of the research study reported.
2. Recognizes common sources of bias in data collection procedures.
3. Interprets data displayed in common types of graphs, charts, or tables.
4. Determines appropriateness of the use of certain common statistical tests.
5. Interprets the stated results of common statistical tests.
6. Obtains the assistance of a professional statistician if the reported statistics are beyond his understanding.
7. Adopts dental procedures judged to be supported by empirical research.

B. *When testing hypotheses of own choosing:*

1. Determines hypothesis.
2. Plans collection of data so that sources of bias are minimized and assumptions of statistical tests will be met.
3. Organizes, summarizes, and displays data in graphs, charts, or tables.
4. Calculates simple statistics.
5. Interprets results.
6. Writes reports on results if deemed appropriate.
7. Obtains assistance of professional statistician if investigation is beyond the scope of his ability.

ILLUSTRATION 3-B

A MINI-CASE: DRUG ABUSE PROBLEMS

INSTRUCTIONAL SITUATION

Dr. Barlowe is planning a course for fourth-year medical students on "Drug Abuse Problems." The professional roles for this course are practicing physicians in different medical specialties. However, the responsibilities of these different specialties regarding drug abuse problems are somewhat different because of the different types of patients seen and the different conditions under which these patients are treated.

QUESTION

Can Dr. Barlowe develop a single list of professional responsibilities that can be used to design a single course appropriate for all his students? If you think so, how should Dr. Barlowe proceed?

FEEDBACK

We think Dr. Barlowe can, in this case, develop a set of responsibilities which are common to all the physician specialties represented by his students. To do this, Dr. Barlowe should first develop a separate list of professional responsibilities for each medical specialty, and then should identify those responsibilities that are common to all or most of these roles. These responsibilities will represent the core of his course, and those responsibilities that are unique to only one role may be dropped or developed into aspects of the course that are optional or assigned as special projects to appropriate students.

DR. BARLOWE'S SOLUTION

I. *Responsibilities of Psychiatrists Regarding Drug Abuse:*

   1. Diagnose and treat drug overdose.
   2. Diagnose withdrawal states and make appropriate disposition.
   3. Prevent, diagnose, and treat psychiatric complications of drug abuse.
   4. Prevent iatrogenic addiction.
   5. Plan and administer drug abuse programs.
   6. Analyze drug abuse literature critically.

II. *Responsibilities of Surgeons Regarding Drug Abuse:*

   1. Prevent, diagnose, and treat surgical complications of drug abuse.
   2. Determine pain medication for drug abuser during postoperative period.
   3. Prevent iatrogenic addiction.
   4. Analyze drug abuse literature critically.
   5. Diagnose and treat drug overdose in emergency situations.
   6. Diagnose withdrawal states and make appropriate disposition, in emergency cases.

III. *Responsibilities of Internists Regarding Drug Abuse:*

   (as above for each of the medical specialties that will be represented by the students)

(Illustration 3-B, continued)

Common Responsibilities

After listing all the responsibilities for each of the medical specialties, Dr. Barlowe was able to identify the following as common to all the future professional roles of his students:

1. Diagnose and treat drug overdose.
2. Diagnose withdrawal states and make appropriate disposition.
3. Prevent, diagnose, treat, or obtain consultation for common complications of drug abuse.
4. Analyze drug abuse literature critically.
5. Prevent iatrogenic addiction.

Responsibilities Unique to Specific Specialties

Dr. Barlowe decided to leave one unit of his course open for students to pursue specific responsibilities related only to their chosen specialty; for example,

Psychiatrists:	Plan and administer drug abuse programs.
Surgeons:	Determine appropriate postoperative pain medication for drug abusers.
Internists:	etc.

ILLUSTRATION 3-C

A MINI-CASE: PSYCHOLOGY

INSTRUCTIONAL SITUATION

The Peabody Nursing School requires that all practical nursing students take a course in psychology during their second year of training. In the past, this course has been taught in the traditional way, that is, a series of lectures and readings covering established topics such as perception, cognition, learning, abnormal behavior, etc. However, students have been complaining that the course is dull, "academic," and not related to nursing.

The Nursing School decided to ask Ms. Klinert to take over this course and redesign it using the model for systematic course design. Ms. Klinert is an experienced nurse who has recently completed a masters in psychology. Identifying the future professional roles was no problem (i.e., practical nurses) but listing professional responsibilities relevant to psychology proved more difficult.

QUESTION

How should Ms. Klinert proceed in developing this list of professional responsibilities?

FEEDBACK

There are several ways Ms. Klinert could approach this problem of an introductory survey course, but none of them are as easy to do as to talk about. The important thing is to focus on ways practical nurses will be able to **use** psychological principles in their daily professional roles. One way to proceed is to locate or develop a detailed list of topics generally dealt with in psychology, and for each topic decide if and how a practical nurse could **use** an underlying principle or skill.

CASE CONTINUED

For example, "perceptual set" is a specific topic under the general topic of perception. Often interpersonal conflicts arise because the different parties have different perceptual sets, that is, they actually perceive different issues because of differences in past experiences, current motives, etc. It would be valuable for a practical nurse to recognize situations when communication has broken down because of such differences in perceptual set. Therefore, an appropriate responsibility related to this topic might be:

> "Recognizes differences in perceptual set as the
> source of interpersonal conflicts and breakdown
> in communication when appropriate."

Examples of other professional responsibilities related to psychology follow:

(Illustration 3-C, continued)

General Topic	*Responsibility*
Learning Theory	• Uses effective techniques when teaching patients to care for themselves.
	• Uses effective techniques to influence patient attitudes toward the hospital, therapeutic adjustments, or life in general.
Growth and Development	• Distinguishes between normal and abnormal behavior in children.
	• Responds appropriately to teenage patients who are struggling with the developmental tasks of adolescence.
Abnormal Behavior	• Recognizes signs of psychological disturbance.
	• Treats disturbed patients with understanding and firmness.

ILLUSTRATION 3-D

A MINI-CASE: PHYSIOLOGY

INSTRUCTIONAL SITUATION

> Dr. Susan Minsky is planning an introductory course in human physiology at a school of public health. The course is available to nonphysician students who have little or no background in biology and are getting advanced degrees in such diversified fields as air pollution control, health services administration, biostatistics, and maternal and child health.

QUESTION 1

Which of the following applies to this course?

    a. It involves multiple future professional roles.

    b. It is an introductory level survey course.

    c. It involves a well-defined subject area that is not easily related to the future professional responsibilities of the students.

    d. It involves teaching someone to teach someone else to do something.

    e. It is an elective course rather than required for some specific set of professional responsibilities.

FEEDBACK

You should have checked all but *d*.

QUESTION 2

How should Dr. Minsky proceed in developing a list of professional responsibilities for her students?

FEEDBACK

Conceivably, Dr. Minsky could develop a set of professional responsibilities for each different professional role by using the steps outlined in Illustration 3-C for an introductory survey course. However, the combination of factors identified in Question 1 above indicates that, in this case, such an extensive analysis may not be worth the effort. That is, it may be better to abandon this portion of the model (i.e., Phase I) and to develop instructional objectives by (a) listing the general topics to be covered, (b) breaking each of these down into specific subtopics, and (c) then deciding what instructional objectives (i.e., terminal student competencies) are appropriate for these specific knowledge areas.

For example, general topics in human physiology include basic cell functions, heredity and cell development, energy metabolism, neural control systems, circulation, etc. One subtopic under the general topic of basic cell functions is "the cell membrane." A possible instructional objective for this specific topic might be: "At the end of this course, students will be able to describe how the cell membrane both protects against bacterial toxins and permits the exchange of nutrients and waste products."

(Illustration 3-D, continued)

A WORD OF CAUTION

Specific instructional objectives developed as described above are likely to be somewhat arbitrary and not necessarily relevant to student needs. However, despite this limitation, it is better to have specific objectives that can be communicated to the students than to have no clear end points at all. Hopefully, the instructor will continually ask himself for each objective written:

- Why do my students need to know this?
- How could they use it in their professional roles?

GUIDELINES FOR SOLVING PROBLEM 3

PROBLEM 3   What if it is difficult to determine professional responsibilities for a subject area?

GUIDELINES   1. If no relevant professional duties come to mind when trying to visualize a competent practitioner in the designated role, then ask yourself:

- **Why** do prospective students need your course at all?
- If students did **not** take your course, where in their professional roles would the deficit show up?

2. If **more than one different professional role** or setting are involved, you may need to:

(a) Analyze each role (or setting) independently to arrive at separate mastery descriptions.
(b) Identify those responsibilities that are common to all or most of the roles (or settings), and
(c) Decide whether to drop those responsibilities that are unique to only one role, or to maintain them as alternate branches within the course.

3. If the course is an **introductory survey** of a broad subject area, then:

(a) Locate or develop a detailed list of topics generally covered in the subject area,
(b) Decide for each topic if and how your students could **use** any underlying concept or skill subsumed under that topic when they assume their professional roles,
(c) Develop responsibilities around potential uses of specific skills or concepts.

4. If the instructional situation involves a combination of problems (such as both multiple roles and survey level coverage of a subject area), consider developing instructional objectives by:

(a) Listing general topics to be covered,
(b) Breaking down general topics into specific subtopics, and
(c) Deciding what you want students to be able to do at the end of your course to demonstrate their mastery of each subtopic.

NOTE: Since this process is likely to lead to arbitrary decisions based on teacher preference rather than on student need, always ask yourself for each objective developed:

- Why do my students need to know this?
- How will they be using it in their professional careers?

PROBLEM 4

How Does One Analyze
The Components Of A Responsibility?

INTRODUCTION It is easy enough to say "now describe the skills, knowledge, and attitudes that are essential in executing each responsibility"; but **doing** this type of analysis is rarely as easy as it appears. In fact, describing the components of the professional responsibilities is the most time-consuming but important task in Phase 1, because it is here that one defines what is actually involved in each responsibility.

The problem in this section is just **how** to determine what these component skills, knowledge, and attitudes ought to be for a specific professional responsibility. That is, how does one begin, how does one know when the job is done, and what steps should one follow to analyze the components of a responsibility?

The materials in this section are designed to **demonstrate** the "thought process" involved in analyzing a professional responsibility, and to provide a general procedure for this process.

DIRECTORY

TYPE OF PROBLEM	RELATED ILLUSTRATION	SEE PAGE
How to proceed	4-A. An Extended Case: Health Care Principles for Day-Care Directors	B-27
Summary	Guidelines for Solving Problem 4	B-37

ILLUSTRATION 4-A

AN EXTENDED CASE: HEALTH CARE PRINCIPLES FOR DAY-CARE DIRECTORS

INSTRUCTIONAL SITUATION

Dr. Kakande is a staff physician at a large city hospital in Africa. She has been asked to teach a one-week course in health care principles for directors of rural day-care centers. This course is the final part of a three-week government-sponsored training program, the first two weeks being devoted to other aspects of operating a day-care center.

About 20 students are expected to attend the program, which will be held at the city hospital where Dr. Kakande works. All students will be female high school graduates who have grown up in the villages where they will operate government-sponsored day-care centers. These centers are sparsely equipped and have limited operating budgets. It is unlikely, for example, that money will be available for feeding or even for equipment such as weight scales.

Dr. Kakande has already specified the responsibilities of these future day-care center directors as related to health care. One of these responsibilities is:

> Recognizes cases of malnutrition.

QUESTION 1

Dr. Kakande is now ready to analyze the skill, knowledge, and attitude components of the above responsibility. The first step is to describe how a competent practitioner would carry out the responsibility in a real-world situation. Which of the following (*a* or *b*) represents the mastery steps involved in recognizing a case of malnutrition that could reasonably be expected of a day-care center director situated in an African village?

    a. (1) Determines growth status on a growth chart by plotting child's weight against age.
       (2) Analyzes blood samples for serum protein and hemoglobin.
       (3) Eliminates possible infections and endocrinologic causes.
    b. (1) Observes children for clinical signs of malnutrition.
       (2) Measures arm circumference.
       (3) Takes diet history if malnutrition is suspected.

FEEDBACK

Although following the steps in *a* is a reliable way to diagnose malnutrition, the day-care directors will *not* have the equipment nor the clinical skill to perform them. The steps listed in *b*, however, represent a mastery performance that can be expected of Dr. Kakande's students.

(Illustration 4-A, continued)

**CASE
CONTINUED**

Dr. Kakande was initially satisfied with the skills she had identified, but as she thought further, she realized that the clinical signs of malnutrition are often ambiguous and could result from other pathological conditions. Likewise, whereas arm circumference is a reasonably effective method for determining fat loss or muscle wasting, it is not totally accurate diagnostically. And diet histories, even if obtained from the child's mother, may not be accurate. Thus, at best, these day-care directors would only be able to identify cases of malnutrition as "probable."

> CAUTION: Changing responsibility ahead!

The process of analyzing a responsibility frequently leads to a change in the specification of the original responsibility. Instead of teaching students to "recognize cases of malnutrition," realistically Dr. Kakande can only teach them to "**identify probable cases of malnutrition**" which could then be referred to a health officer for verification. Although this new wording of the responsibility may seem trivial, it states the real-world situation more precisely, thus giving Dr. Kakande a better idea of where her course must aim.

**SUMMARY OF
PROGRESS**

Thus far Dr. Kakande has decided that the skill components involved in this responsibility include:

(1) observing children for clinical signs,
(2) measuring arm circumference, and
(3) taking a diet history.

**CASE
CONTINUED**

It is evident that to look for clinical signs, one must know what these signs are. Thus these clinical signs should be listed as knowledge components. Here is how Dr. Kakande began to enumerate the clinical signs of malnutrition:

"Let's see now, there's depigmentation of the hair, muscular wasting, enlarged abdomen . . . but that could also be worms . . . and then there is rickets caused by Vitamin D deficiency . . . hmmm . . ."

As she recalled these clinical signs, Dr. Kakande realized how complex the diagnosis really is. Not only do some signs sometimes indicate **other** clinical conditions, but there are several different types of malnutrition. What should be specified as the necessary knowledge components for these students?

(Illustration 4-A, continued)

Whenever the subject matter is complex, one must determine what is reasonable and feasible for students to learn within the constraints of the course. In this case, Dr. Kakande must decide if her students will need to identify the different types of malnutrition or if it will be sufficient for them to recognize only the most common or most important types of malnutrition. Likewise, she must decide if her students need to know what other conditions manifest the same clinical signs as does malnutrition.

It is never easy to decide what students actually "need to know" in relation to what feasibly can be taught, and rarely are there any clearly "right" or "wrong" decisions. One must simply decide and move on.

QUESTION 2   Dr. Kakande decided that because **protein calorie malnutrition** was the most common and important form of malnutrition, she would concentrate on that. Having decided once more to restrict the subject area, what should she do next?

 a. Change the responsibility again—this time to "identify probable cases of protein calorie malnutrition (PCM)."
 b. Edit skill and knowledge components already listed so that they involve only PCM.
 c. Both of the above.

FEEDBACK   Whenever one changes the scope of a responsibility, it is important not only to change the wording of the responsibility but also to review all parts of the analysis of components to determine the extent of revision necessary.

SUMMARY OF PROGRESS   After the clinical signs were added to the knowledge components, the analysis looked like this:

SKILLS	KNOWLEDGE
1. Observes children for one or more clinical signs.	(1) Clinical signs of PCM: a. marked weakness b. skinny arms and legs c. pot belly (could also be worms) d. puffy eyes, face, arms, or legs e. hair color changes from black to reddish-brown.
2. Measures arm circumference. 3. Takes a diet history.	

(Illustration 4-A, continued)

CASE CONTINUED

At this point Dr. Kakande realized that the skills she had listed were **not** specific enough to clarify the **process** involved in identifying a probable case of PCM. For example, to "observe a child for clinical signs," one must examine particular aspects of the child; and "measuring arm circumference" involves a series of discrete steps. So she decided to spell out each of these procedures in more detail.

By referring to the knowledge components she had already listed, Dr. Kakande discovered that "observing children for clinical signs" involves examining:

(a) the child's general energy level;
(b) the condition of the arms, legs, belly and face; and
(c) the color of the hair.

When she thought about the process involved in measuring arm circumference, Dr. Kakande realized that the problem here is locating the proper site for taking the measurement, since taking a measurement too low or too high invalidates this screening test. The day-care director must be able to locate the **midpoint** of a child's upper arm. That is done by measuring the total distance from the depression at the tip of the shoulder bone to the tip of the elbow, and then taking half of this distance and marking the child's arm. If the circumference at this site is 12 cm or less, then the child's arm is in the lower 3% range for children aged 2-5, which is dangerously low and indicates fat loss and/or marked wasting. But, again, for this 12-cm-cutoff point to be meaningful, the child's arm must be relaxed at his or her side.

Dr. Kakande was surprised that this "simple" arm circumference test involved so many details once she started thinking about them. Yet this is often the case whenever the specific skills of any procedure are analyzed. The important point here, however, is that after thinking through the steps and potential problems in this way, usually one can then summarize and later teach the process sequentially and succinctly.

(Illustration 4-A, continued)

SUMMARY OF PROGRESS

When Dr. Kakande finished specifying the skills, her analysis looked like this (notice that she added a final step after working out the details of the first three):

SKILLS	KNOWLEDGE
1. *Observes children* for one or more signs. Look specifically at: — general energy level — condition of arms, legs, belly, and face — color of the hair 2. *Measures arm circumference* to determine if lower than standard. a. have child bend arm at elbow b. locate midpoint of upper arm c. have child relax arm at side d. determine if circumference at midpoint is 12 cm or less 3. *Takes diet history* from mother or sibling who comes to pick up child. Ask: — if child is growing as well as others in family — what foods child eats/likes — how "well" child eats 4. *Decides* whether to report a given child to local health officer as probable case of PCM.	(1) *Clinical signs of PCM:* a. marked weakness or inactivity b. skinny arms and legs c. pot belly (could also be worms) d. puffy eyes, face, arms, or legs e. hair color changes from black to reddish-brown

CASE CONTINUED

To complete the knowledge components, one should look at each of the skills and ask: "What does the day-care director need to **know** to perform this skill?" For example, to perform the arm circumference test, these students may need to know more about how and why the test works. That is, they need to know that the upper arm is made of a bone wrapped in muscle, fat, and skin; that the narrowest place on this bone is the midpoint; and that a circumference measurement at this midpoint of 12 cm or less indicates serious fat loss and possibly muscular wasting.

(Illustration 4-A, continued)

QUESTION 3   Which items below represent knowledge components you think are necessary for skill 3, "Takes diet history from mother or siblings who come to pick up child"?

    a. What foods in the village diet are major sources of protein and calories.
    b. How food is digested.
    c. How protein and calorie deficiencies create the various clinical signs.
    d. That diet information obtained this way is only a gross indicator.

FEEDBACK   Dr. Kakande chose items *a* and *d*. Items *b* and *c* are related to the general topic but are **not** essential knowledge for performing this behavior. That is, to take a diet history one does **not** need to understand how food is digested or how each clinical sign develops.

QUESTION 4   What are the knowledge components of skill 4? That is, after completing skills 1, 2, and 3, what must someone know to "decide whether to report a given child to the local health officer"?

FEEDBACK   Dr. Kakande developed the following knowledge components for this step:

Criteria for decision: Any one or combination of

    (a) the clinical signs,
    (b) arm circumference 12cm or less,
    (c) suspicion that child is not eating sufficient P and C.

CASE
CONTINUED   After considering each skill individually as above, it is a good idea to review the responsibility as a whole to determine if any important components have been omitted. In this case, Dr. Kakande decided her students should know the usual stages in the development of PCM, beginning with inadequate intake of protein and calories and ending with the manifest clinical signs. She considered this important theoretical knowledge, since students should have some idea how far a case may have progressed before its detection.

SUMMARY
OF PROGRESS   The analysis of the responsibility now looks as follows:

(Illustration 4-A, continued)

Responsibility: Identifies probable cases of protein calorie malnutrition (PCM).

SKILLS	KNOWLEDGE
1. *Observes children* for one or more clinical signs. Look specifically at: — general energy level — condition of arms, legs, belly, and face — color of the hair.	(1) *Clinical signs of PCM:* a. marked weakness or inactivity b. skinny arms and legs c. pot belly (could also be worms) d. puffy eyes, face, arms or legs e. hair color changes from black to reddish-brown.
2. *Measures arm circumference* to determine if lower than standard: a. has child bend arm at elbow b. locates midpoint of upper arm c. has child relax arm at side d. determines if circumference at midpoint is 12cm or less.	(2) *How arm circumference test works:* — upper arm made of a bone wrapped in muscle, fat, and skin — narrowest place on bone is midpoint — 12cm or less indicates serious fat loss and/or muscle wasting.
3. *Takes diet history* from mother or sibling who comes to pick up child. Ask: — if child is growing as well as others in family — what foods child eats/likes — how "well" the child eats.	(3) *Major sources of protein and calories* in the foods eaten in village (diet information obtained in this way is rarely accurate; only a very gross indicator).
4. *Decides whether to report* a given child to local health officer as a probable case of PCM.	(4) *Criteria for decision:* Any one or combination of: a. presence of clinical sign(s) b. arm circumference 12cm or less c. suspicion that child not eating sufficient P and C. *Background Theory*—Sequence of events resulting in PCM: inadequate nutritional intake → loss of fat → muscle wasting → one or more clinical signs.

B-33

(Illustration 4-A, continued)

CASE CONTINUED

Having determined the skill and knowledge components of the responsibility, Dr. Kakande turned to the issue of attitude components: Are there any desirable values or general styles that would be helpful for day-care center directors in carrying out this responsibility?

The first thing that occurred to Dr. Kakande was that her students must become aware of the seriousness of the malnutrition problem in these rural villages. Hopefully if they realize how prevalent the disease is and the consequences of failing to treat it, they will be more attentive in watching for clinical signs. So, across from the skill "observes children for one or more clinical signs," Dr. Kakande wrote:

> "(1) Awareness of the prevalence of PCM and
> consequences of failing to treat it."

QUESTION 5

Is there an important attitude or style for a day-care director to have while performing the second skill, that is, "measuring arm circumference to determine if lower than standard"? For example, how should one handle the child during such a procedure?

FEEDBACK

Dr. Kakande thought it was important to handle the child gently so as not to frighten him or her. Also, it would be helpful to talk to the child but **not** to alarm the child with the reason for the test.

QUESTION 6

Can you think of important attitudes related to the third and fourth skill components, that is, "taking a diet history from the mother or sibling" and "deciding whether to report a child to local health officer"? **Note**: It is **not** necessary to have an attitude component for **every** skill.

FEEDBACK

Certainly the taking of a diet history must be done with the appropriate tone—casual and nonthreatening. Village mothers or siblings will probably want to please, and if they sense it is important to give particular answers, they will; and the resulting information may be biased accordingly.

Dr. Kakande could not think of any critical attitude component associated with the fourth skill, and thus left it blank.

SUMMARY OF PROGRESS

Once she had filled in the third column with attitude components, the analysis of the responsibility looked as follows:

(Illustration 4-A, continued)

Course Title: Health Care Principles
for Day-Care Directors

ANALYZED RESPONSIBILITY

Responsibility: Identifies probable cases of protein calorie malnutrition (PCM)

SKILLS	KNOWLEDGE	ATTITUDES
1. *Observes children* for one or more clinical signs. Looks at: — general energy level — condition of arms, legs, belly, and face — color of the hair.	(1) *Clinical signs of PCM:* a. marked weakness or inactivity b. skinny arms and legs c. pot belly (could also be worms) d. puffy eyes, face, arms, or legs e. hair color changes from black to reddish brown.	(1) Awareness of prevalence of PCM and consequences of failing to treat it.
2. *Measures arm circumference* to determine if lower than standard: a. has child bend arm at elbow b. locates midpoint of upper arm c. has child relax arm at side d. determines if circumference at midpoint is 12cm or less.	(2) *How arm circumference test works:* — Upper arm is made of a bone wrapped in muscle, fat and skin — Narrowest place on bone is midpoint — 12cm or less indicates serious fat loss and/or muscle wasting.	(2) Handles and talks to child gently so as not to alarm him or her.
3. *Takes diet history* from mother or sibling who comes to pick up child. Asks: — if child is growing as well as others in the family — what foods child eats/likes — how "well" the child eats.	(3) *Major sources of protein and calories* in the foods eaten in village (diet information obtained in this way is rarely accurate; only a gross indicator).	(3) Questions mother or sibling in a casual nonthreatening way.
4. *Decides* whether to report a given child to local health officer as a probable case of PCM.	(4) *Criteria for decisions:* Any one or combination of: a. presence of clinical signs(s) b. arm circumference of 12cm or less c. suspicion that child not eating sufficient protein and calories. Background Theory—Sequence of events resulting in PCM: inadequate nutritional intake → loss of fat → muscle wasting → one or more clinical signs.	

(Illustration 4-A, continued)

CASE CONTINUED	After completing the skill, knowledge, and attitude components as above, Dr. Kakande was satisfied that if daycare directors could learn to do and know these things, they would be able to discharge this responsibility related to malnutrition. However, in reviewing the entire analysis once again, she discovered an inconsistency between the **stated** responsibility and what she actually wanted students to do, as indicated by the specified skills. As a result of this discovery, she revised the wording of the responsibility once again.
QUESTION 7	Can you locate the inconsistency between the stated responsibility and the skills outlined above? How would you edit the responsibility so it adequately describes the **intended** performance?
FEEDBACK	Dr. Kakande wants her students to do more than "identify" probable cases of PCM, she wants them to "refer" these children to their local health officers. A more precise way to state the responsibility, then, would be:

"Identifies probable cases of PCM for
referral to local health officers."

(End of Case)

GUIDELINES FOR SOLVING PROBLEM 4

PROBLEM 4

How does one analyze the components of a responsibility? That is, how does one determine what skills, knowledge, and attitudes to specify for a given responsibility?

GUIDELINES

1. *Determine skill components* by imagining you are observing a competent practitioner carry out the responsibility in the real world. Write down each step he or she would perform.

   a. Use **action verbs** for every skill you list, since you are describing performance.
   b. Be **specific** enough to clarify the process involved in each step or skill.
   c. If the analysis changes your thinking regarding the scope of the responsibility, **modify** accordingly.
   d. Don't forget to include such component skills as:

      — recognizing **when** to perform an activity
      — deciding what action to take
      — planning an approach to take
      — selecting equipment
      — locating materials
      — evaluating one's own performance.

2. *Determine knowledge components* by examining each skill component and deciding what, if anything, someone must "know" to perform this behavior in the real world. Describe these knowledge components in as much detail as seems reasonable.

   a. If knowledge components are associated with a particular skill, display and/or code them to illustrate this relationship.
   b. Limit the knowledge components to those you intend to include in the course. Some details may be "nice-to-know," but not essential for your course.
   c. Be sure to include such knowledge components as:

      — technical vocabulary
      — criteria for decisions
      — underlying facts, concepts or theory
      — difference between a proper and improper performance.

3. *Determine attitude components* by reviewing each component skill once again and deciding if there are any desirable values or general approaches toward one's self, work, or others which would facilitate the execution of that component skill or the entire responsibility.

a. Do **not** feel you **must** develop an attitude component for every skill component.

b. When appropriate, display and/or code attitude components to illustrate their relationship to specific skills.

c. Consider including such attitudes as:

- awareness of the **importance** of the responsibility or component skill
- awareness of consequences or dangers of **not** performing the responsibility or skill
- desire to perform according to some standard.

PROBLEM 5

What If It Is Difficult To Analyze Components Of A Responsibility?

INTRODUCTION   Often the process of analyzing responsibilities uncovers various problems related to organization, level of detail, and consistency, etc. Many of the decisions that must be made to solve these problems will be arbitrary on the part of the instructor, but certain guidelines may be helpful.

Typical reasons for having difficulty analyzing a responsibility include:

(a) The differences between skill, knowledge and attitude components may be ambiguous.

(b) The skill components may *not* be equivalent in scope (i.e. step size).

(c) The responsibility may be too broad in scope, or too specific.

(d) The "responsibility" may actually be a knowledge or attitude component of some other responsibility.

The materials in this section demonstrate each of these types of problems and provide opportunities to practice solving them.

DIRECTORY

TYPE OF PROBLEM	RELATED ILLUSTRATION	SEE PAGE
Distinguishing between skill, knowledge, and attitude components	5-A. A Feedback Exercise: Performing a White Blood Cell Count	B-40
Skills not equivalent in scope	5-B. A Mini-Case: Immunization	B-42
Scope of responsibility too broad or specific	5-C. A Feedback Exercise: Levels of Detail	B-45
"Responsibility" actually a knowledge or attitude component	5-D. A Feedback Exercise: Recognizing Components	B-48
Summary	Guidelines for Solving Problem 5	B-50

ILLUSTRATION 5-A

A FEEDBACK EXERCISE:
PERFORMING A WHITE CELL COUNT

INTRODUCTION	Sometimes teachers have difficulty analyzing the components of a responsibility because they fail to distinguish accurately between skills, knowledge, and attitudes.
DIRECTIONS	Below is a scrambled list of components for the responsibility "Performs a white blood cell count." First decide whether each component is a **skill**, **knowledge**, or **attitude**. Then decide which knowledge components should be associated with which skill components.
SCRAMBLED LIST	a. Be meticulous about accuracy. b. Appropriate level to which to draw blood in pipette. c. For accuracy, chamber must be full but not overflowing. d. Fills counting chamber with specimen. e. Draws blood into clean dry pipette to correct mark. f. Appreciates the importance of accuracy for assisting in correct clinical interpretation of patient's problem. g. Cleans pipette(s) and counting chamber(s). h. Range of normal white blood cell count. i. Interprets resulting count and repeats entire procedure if outside range of normal. j. Counts white cells under microscope. k. Correction formula and its rationale. l. Characteristics both of white cells and of artifacts to avoid in count. m. Corrects resulting count. n. Mixes blood with diluent by rotating pipette. o. Draws diluent into pipette to correct mark. p. How long and vigorously to rotate pipette. q. Appropriate level to which to draw diluent.
FEEDBACK	Skills: *d, e, g, i, j, m, n,* and *o.* Knowledge: *b, c, h, k, l, p,* and *q.* Attitudes: *a* and *f.* In the following table these components are arranged in their proper sequence and relationship to each other.

(Illustration 5-A, continued)

<table>
<tr><td colspan="3" align="right">Course Title: Laboratory Procedures</td></tr>
<tr><td colspan="3" align="center">**ANALYZED RESPONSIBILITY**</td></tr>
<tr><td colspan="3">Responsibility: Performs a white blood cell count.</td></tr>
<tr><td align="center">SKILLS</td><td align="center">KNOWLEDGE</td><td align="center">ATTITUDE</td></tr>
<tr>
<td>

1. Draws blood into clean dry pipette to correct mark.

2. Draws diluent into pipette to correct mark.

3. Mixes blood with diluent by rotating pipette.

4. Fills counting chamber with specimen.

5. Counts white cells under microscope.

6. Corrects resulting count.

7. Interprets resulting count and repeats entire procedure if outside range of normal.

8. Cleans pipette(s) and counting chamber(s)

</td>
<td>

(1) Appropriate level to which to draw blood in pipette

(2) Appropriate level to which to draw diluent

(3) How long and vigorously to rotate pipette

(4) For accuracy, chamber must be full but not overflowing

(5) Characteristics both of white cells and of artifacts to avoid

(6) Correction formula and its rationale

(7) Range of normal white blood cell count

</td>
<td>

(For all steps in the procedure)

(a) Be meticulous about accuracy.

(b) Appreciate the importance of accuracy for assisting in correct clinical interpretation of patient's problem

</td>
</tr>
</table>

ILLUSTRATION 5-B

A MINI-CASE: IMMUNIZATION

INSTRUCTIONAL SITUATION

Dr. Josefs is teaching a course on immunization for medical assistants in Africa. Each medical assistant will eventually hold a responsible position in a village or community in rural Africa.

One of the professional responsibilities for this position is "Identifies those individuals within their area who need immunization." The analysis Dr. Josefs developed for this responsibility is shown on page B-43.

After he finished this analysis, Dr. Josefs realized that skill component 2 involved considerably more content and was broader in scope than any of the other skill components. Gaining access to the target population is a major activity that includes teaching the community about immunization.

QUESTION

What, if anything, should Dr. Josefs do?

    a. Revise the analysis by describing skill component 2 in more detail or by dividing it into two or three additional skill components.

    b. Create a new responsibility for skill 2 and analyze it separately.

    c. Nothing. As long as Dr. Josefs knows what is involved in skill 2, he doesn't need to write it out.

FEEDBACK

Since he believed that teaching the community the advantages of immunization was an important but often overlooked responsibility of medical assistants, Dr. Josefs decided to create a new responsibility and to analyze it separately, as is shown on page B-44. However, a different instructor may have preferred one of the other alternatives, depending on the amount of emphasis to be given to skill component 2 during the course itself. The first alternative (revise by describing skill 2 in more detail) is probably **less** desirable than the third (do nothing), since the details of skill 2 are *not* closely related to the other skills or to the responsibility as stated.

(Illustration 5-B, continued)

	Course Title: Immunization for Medical Assistants

ANALYZED RESPONSIBILITY

Responsibility: Identifies individuals who need immunization.

SKILLS	KNOWLEDGE	ATTITUDES

1. Identifies target population:
  a. Determines eligible ages.
  b. Identifies high risk groups.
	Definitions:
	  – target population
	  – high-risk group.
		Understands the importance of immunization for a community.

2. Gains access to target population:
  a. Contacts community institutions.
  b. Gives health education talks.
  c. Screens clients coming to health center.
	What a community needs to know about immunization.	

3. Determines if immunization is needed by individuals:
  a. Determines age.
  b. Checks for previous immunizations (look for scars, ask mother, etc).
  c. Recalls immunization schedule to decide if immunization is needed.
	Regular immunization schedule including:
	  – ages for each vaccine
	  – target diseases
	  – characteristics of different vaccines.
		Appreciates the value of having and using an immunization schedule.

4. Considers contraindications:
  a. Recalls contraindications.
  b. Checks for presence of those contraindications in patient and his family.
  c. Excludes if contraindications are present.
	Contraindications for each different vaccine:
	  – nature of contraindication
	  – how to deal with it.
	
	Background Theory:
	  – Responses of an organism to an infectious agent
	  – Ways to protect organism:
	    a. isolation
	    b. passive or active immunization.
		Realizes the seriousness of these contraindications if not discovered.

(Illustration 5-B, continued)

Course Title: Immunization for
Medical Assistants

ANALYZED RESPONSIBILITY

Responsibility: Teaches the advantages of immunization to the community

SKILLS	KNOWLEDGE	ATTITUDES

1. Finds occasions to teach:
  a. Looks for existing situations that allow for teaching.
  b. Creates situations that allow teaching.
	– Types of existing situations to look for (e.g., political, educational, or community service groups).
	– Types of situations where people could be invited for health talks.
		Exhibit genuine interest; do **not** be condescending.

2. Ascertains people's attitudes toward immunization:
  a. Determines what they believe.
  b. Asks about past experiences.
  c. Asks if they would get immunizations for selves and for children, and if not, why.
	– An attitude is a predisposition toward action based on one's beliefs and memories.
	– Methods for determining attitudes such as interviews, questionnaires, rating scales, etc.	

3. Plans teaching approaches for
  – formal presentations, and
  – the unexpected individual encounter.		

4. Describes benefits from immunization:
  a. Compares occurrence and effects of infectious diseases with and without immunization.
  b. Discusses diseases that can be prevented but not effectively treated once they occur.
	– Effects of immunization on disease
	Individual: prevents or decreases seriousness
	Community: reduces incidence and possibly eradicates
	– Diseases which can be prevented but not treated effectively once they occur.
		Set an appropriate climate for communication (watch for signs of confusion; treat all questions as important, etc).

5. Points out that advantages of immunization are possible only if entire community cooperates.	– Why only immunization of large numbers can protect the whole community.	
6. Tries to deal with any negative attitudes.	– Typical negative attitudes and ways to counter them.	Be respectful and tolerant; never belittle these negative attitudes.

ILLUSTRATION 5-C

A FEEDBACK EXERCISE: LEVELS OF DETAIL

INTRODUCTION

Sometimes a "responsibility" turns out to be either too broad or too specific to be analyzed conveniently or taught as a cohesive unit of instruction. The broader the scope of a responsibility, the larger the size of each component skill; that is, the more behaviors (discrete actions) are encompassed by each step of the procedure.

Below a broad responsibility has been broken down into several levels of detail (or smaller sizes of steps).

Level 1	Level 2	Level 3	Level 4
		(a) Administers anesthesia	(1) Selects needle
			(2) Selects anesthesia
			(3) Selects injection site
		(b) Selects instruments	(4) Prepares needle
			(5) Prepares site
	1. Extracts teeth	(c) Inserts elevators	(6) Gives injection
Treats common dental problems	2. Fills cavities	(d) Performs forceps extraction	
	3. Relieves pain	(e) Performs post-extraction care	
	4. Scales teeth		

QUESTION 1

At which level of detail above should one write professional responsibilities and which level(s) should be included in the analysis of components?

— —

FEEDBACK

The above question has no single answer. In general the behavior described by the responsibility should be broken down during the analysis of that responsibility into at least one, and often two, more detailed levels. However, the appropriate level of detail for the responsibility itself depends in part on the size and scope of the intended instructional unit. The smaller the scope of the instruction, the more useful it is to specify the responsibilities in greater detail.

QUESTION 2

Which of the following has a broader instructional scope?

a. An introductory course on simple dental procedures for medical assistants in rural South America.

b. An advanced seminar on the administration of anesthesia for third-year dental students.

— —

(Illustration 5-C, continued)

FEEDBACK   The introductory course has the broader instructional scope. Relevant professional responsibilities for these medical assistants should probably be stated at the second level shown on the diagram above. These then would be broken down during the analysis into levels 3 and 4. On the other hand, responsibilities for the advanced seminar on anesthesia would probably be written at Level 4 of the diagram, and their analyses would involve additional details at Levels 5 and perhaps 6 (not shown in the diagram).

COMMENT   Although the level of specificity will vary as a function of the scope of the course being developed, to a large extent step-size is a matter of personal preference. However, as you select a level of detail for your own responsibilities, the following might be helpful:

1. Generally, the more specific the responsibilities, the easier it is to design and evaluate the instruction. It takes more time to develop and analyze responsibilities in greater detail, but during that process the instructor determines the content of the course and clarifies what is expected of the students.
2. On the other hand, since analyzing a responsibility involves breaking it down into additional levels of detail, the analysis could result in trivial substeps if the responsibility is already too specific.

QUESTION 3   First, decide whether each of the following is (a) probably too broad, (b) probably too specific, or (c) probably about right for responsibilities of nurses (regarding general nursing school courses). Then decide what should be done about those that are too broad or too specific.

1. Records dates of immunizations.
2. Gives nutritional advice to mothers.
3. Administers injections.
4. Diagnoses and treats 20 common childhood ailments.
5. Supervises ward activites.
6. Disposes of used bandages.
7. Cleans wounds and changes dressings.

FEEDBACK   1. *Probably too specific.* Recording the date of an immunization is probably a component skill of a responsibility such as "performs immunizations" or "maintains records of immunizations," either of which would involve additional component skills.

2. *Probably about right.* Conceivably an entire course could be built around this one responsibility, but within the context of the usual nursing school

(Illustration 5-C, continued)

courses, giving nutritional advice to mothers is a reasonable block of instructional content for one responsibility.

3. *Probably about right.* Giving injections is an important responsibility of nurses and one that involves a number of important behaviors, but none of which are excessively complex.

4. *Probably too broad.* Unless some of these childhood ailments can be grouped into categories, it may be necessary here to create 20 different responsibilities, one for each ailment.

5. *Probably too broad.* A number of complex management skills are involved in supervising a ward, including planning work schedules, making assignments, monitoring progress, disciplining employees, maintaining records, etc. Unless the curriculum de-emphasizes these management skills, each probably merits a separate responsibility.

6. *Probably too specific.* Disposing of used bandages is probably a component skill of the responsibility "changes bandages."

7. *Probably too broad.* It would probably be easier to handle the cleaning of a wound and the changing of a dressing in separate responsibilities. However, since they are clearly related, conceivably some instructors would prefer to analyze and handle them together.

ILLUSTRATION 5-D

A FEEDBACK EXERCISE: RECOGNIZING COMPONENTS

INTRODUCTION

Sometimes a "responsibility" doesn't appear to have any component skills at all, or at least they are not immediately apparent. When this happens, the original "responsibility" often turns out **not** to be a true responsibility but is rather a knowledge or attitude component of some other responsibility.

EXAMPLE 1 (KNOWLEDGE COMPONENT)

Original Responsibility:

(for environmental health specialist)

Understands the meteorologic aspects (e.g., air currents, storms, etc.) of the transmission of air pollutants from source to man.

There are no skill components involved in "understanding" something, because understanding implies knowledge, not performance. To determine the responsibility of which this is a knowledge component, one should ask **why** students need to understand these meteorologic aspects. How will they **use** this knowledge? In this case, environmental health specialists need to understand these aspects of air pollution so that they can select appropriate control measures for specific air pollutants.

Revised Responsibility:

Selects appropriate control measures for specific air pollutants.

EXAMPLE 2 (ATTITUDE COMPONENT)

Original Responsibility:

(for physician)

Treats all patients with respect.

Everyone would agree that this is a very important and often neglected aspect of a physician's profession. However, treating patients with respect involves a basic approach or attitude toward patients that is manifested every time the physician interacts with a patient. As such, this is an attitude component of every professional responsibility which involves patient interaction, such as taking histories, performing physical examinations, etc.

(Illustration 5-D, continued)

QUESTION

First decide whether each of the following "responsibilities" actually involves an attitude or knowledge. Then determine what true responsibility each should be a component of by asking:

(For knowledge components)
- Why do students need to know this?
- What will they be doing when they use this knowledge/understanding?

(For attitudes components)
- When will students exhibit this attitude?
- What will they be doing when they manifest this attitude?

Original "Responsibilities"

a. Works carefully but efficiently (for lab technician).

b. Understands the political issues involved in hospital management (for nurse).

c. Understands the roles of dental hygienists, assistants, and technicians (for dentist).

d. Appreciates the importance of notifying public health officials of all cases of reportable infectious diseases (for physician).

FEEDBACK

a. This **attitude** component should probably be part of every responsibility of the lab technician.

b. Nurses probably need some understanding of hospital politics to operate effectively within such an environment. An appropriate responsibility for this **knowledge** component might be "operates effectively in the political atmosphere of a hospital." Component skills would then consist of behaviors such as: recognizes political issues behind management decisions, identifies sources of political pressures, reports problems to appropriate personnel, etc.

c. Dentists need to understand the roles of these ancillary dental personnel to use them effectively in their practices. Thus an appropriate responsibility to be analyzed in this case would be "utilizes ancillary dental personnel effectively."

d. Appreciating the importance of something is probably an attitude, but some consider this a knowledge component. Certainly the **reasons** for something being important are knowledge components, but what is really at stake here is the "feeling" that something is vital. At any rate, the responsibility to be analyzed should be "notifies public health officials of all cases of reportable infectious diseases."

GUIDELINES FOR SOLVING PROBLEM 5

PROBLEM 5   What if it is difficult to analyze the skill, knowledge, and attitude components of a responsibility?

SPECIFIC PROBLEM	POSSIBLE EXPLANATION	SUGGESTED GUIDELINES
Skills not equivalent in scope	One or more skills may be entire responsibilities by themselves.	Convert oversized skills into new responsibilities and analyze their components independently.
Too many skill and/or knowledge components	May be too broad in scope for a single responsibility.	Divide into several smaller responsibilities and analyze each independently.
Too few skill and/or knowledge components	May be too specific for a responsibility; that is, it may be a component skill of some other responsibility.	Incorporate as a skill component of a related broader responsibility.
Does not seem to have had skill components	May be a knowledge or attitude component of some other responsibility.	Incorporate as a knowledge or attitude component of the appropriate responsibility. Determine appropriate responsibility by asking **why** and **when** someone would need to know this or to manifest this attitude.

PROBLEM 6

Why Choose One Method Of Performance Analysis Over Another?

INTRODUCTION   After the **optimal** professional performance has been described, it is important to validate this mastery description by analyzing **actual** professional performance. A number of performance analysis methods are available for this purpose, but it is not always easy to decide which is most appropriate for a given instructional situation.

The materials in this section are designed to give practice and guidelines in selecting methods of performance analysis.

NOTE: Before continuing with this section, read or review Chapter 7 in Unit C of this book (beginning on page C-5), which describes the various methods of performance analysis considered in this section.

DIRECTORY

TYPE OF PROBLEM	RELATED ILLUSTRATION	SEE PAGE
How to determine appropriate method of performance an- analysis	6-A. A Feedback Exercise: selecting methods of performance analysis	B-52
Summary	Guidelines for Solving Problem 6	B-55

ILLUSTRATION 6-A

A FEEDBACK EXERCISE: SELECTING METHODS OF PERFORMANCE ANALYSIS

INTRODUCTION   In general, reasons for selecting one method of performance analysis over another involve criteria such as:

(a) the number, location, and availability of existing practitioners and/or experts in the subject area,

(b) the extent to which the responsibilities are readily observable in actual practice,

(c) the level of expertise and previous experience of the instructor, and

(d) the amount of time available both to the instructor and to the practitioners and/or subject matter experts.

QUESTION   Each of the course titles listed below refers to a mini-case previously described on the page indicated in parentheses. Review the instructional situation and known responsibilities for each mini-case and then decide which of the following methods of performance analysis would be particularly *appropriate* and which would probably be *inappropriate*, and why.

Methods of Performance Analysis

1. Questionnaire
2. Critical incident technique
3. Log diary
4. Checklist
5. Observation interview
6. Work participation
7. Individual interview
8. Group interview
9. Technical conference

Mini-Cases

a. Utilization of Community Resources, for practicing physicians (see Illustration 2-A, page B-13).

b. Performing a White Blood Cell Count, for lab technicians (see Illustration 5-A, page B-40).

c. Psychology, for practical nurses (see Illustration 3-C, page B-21).

(Illustration 6-A, continued)

d. Immunization, for medical assistants (see Illustration 5-B, page B-42).

e. Tropical Medicine, for directors of public health programs, research scientists, teachers, and private practitioners (see Illustration 1-A, page B-7).

————————————————————————————————————

FEEDBACK

a. UTILIZATION OF COMMUNITY RESOURCES

There are three sources of subject matter expertise related to this course: (1) currently practicing physicians who are now utilizing community resources particularly well, (2) individuals who direct or work in various community service agencies, and (3) patients who in the past have been referred to these community resources by physicians. Personnel from the community agencies are probably the best place to begin, since they would be the best source for locating physicians and patients who have used the referral system. *Individual* or, preferably, *group interviews* with such personnel might be solicited from these persons during such interviews. If the directors of these community resources wanted to or had the time to participate more directly in the course being developed, a *technical conference* might be set up which would also include consumers and physicians. Otherwise, experienced patients could be polled for *critical incidents*, and *individual interviews* could be conducted with physicians identified as particularly good at utilizing community resources. Conceivably an *observation interview* could also be involved if such a physician had a good filing system, or patients needing referral reasonably often. The *log diary, checklist,* and *work participation* methods would probably **not** be appropriate for any of the subject matter experts, since the responsibilities involved here are performed intermittently amidst other activities.

b. PERFORMING A WHITE BLOOD CELL COUNT

Since this is a rather simple, technical procedure, the *checklist, observation interview,* or *work participation* methods could be applied most appropriately, depending on the practicing lab technicians who could be solicited to serve as subject matter experts, and on the needs of the instructor. For example, the instructor may need the experience of working in a lab, or may need to question the person being observed in order to understand everything that is done. A *technical conference* or *group interview* would probably **not** be necessary here. *Questionnaires* could be used (or better yet the *critical incident technique*) if actual observation could not be arranged. A *log diary* is probably **not** appropriate, but might be used to get information on timing.

(Illustration 6-A, continued)

c. PSYCHOLOGY

Analyzing actual professional performance in this case is going to be almost as difficult as describing it. Subject matter experts that conceivably could be used are (1) practicing nurses, (2) previous students, (3) medical sociologists, and (4) members of the school's curriculum committee. The most appropriate methods to use include the *critical incident technique, group interview,* and *technical conference. Checklist, work participation,* and *observation interviews* are probably out of the question. *Questionnaires* or *individual interviews* might be used, but not as a first choice.

d. IMMUNIZATION

The method to be used here depends heavily on who are available as subject matter experts. The instructor may not have the time or money available to travel to distant rural areas to *interview* or *observe* currently practicing medical assistants. This type of experience, however, should be the first choice. Possibly in the urban center where the course is being taught, Dr. Josefs could locate several past-medical assistants or, at least, individuals who have had some experience working in rural areas. Individuals who organize and supervise the activities of medical assistants for an entire region might also serve as subject matter experts. *Questionnaires* with *log diaries* sent to currently practicing medical assistants could be used if direct interviewing is not possible. Collecting *critical incidents* from practitioners or any persons involved in the system would be helpful. The *group interview* or *technical conference* would be good but may not be easy to arrange.

e. TROPICAL MEDICINE

Here we have a case of multiple roles—so whatever methods are used, an attempt must be made to include at least the most important of these roles. A *questionnaire* to previous students is an excellent method for such a course. *Critical incidents* could be solicited as part of this questionnaire, but *log diaries* would probably add only extraneous information. *Individual interviews* could be conducted with knowledgeable persons, such as departmental colleagues or individuals who have in the past held positions as directors of public health programs in tropical countries. If these same individuals could be collected in one place at one time, a *group interview* or *technical conference* would also be appropriate. Inappropriate techniques include the *checklist, observation interview,* and *work participation* methods, because the responsibilities do not lend themselves readily to observation.

GUIDELINES FOR SOLVING PROBLEM 6

PROBLEM 6

Why choose. one method of performance analysis over another for a particular instructional situation?

GUIDELINES

1. Determine **what subject matter experts** are available. Existing competent practitioners? Previous practitioners? Supervisors of practitioners? Consumers or patients? Experts in the subject area?

2. Decide the best way to obtain the most useful information from available experts.

   a. If it is possible for you to observe or try out certain procedures in a real setting, consider the **checklist, observation interview,** or **work participation methods.**

   b. If the experts could be gathered in one place at one time, and would benefit from the group interaction, consider the **group interview** or **technical conference** methods.

   c. Collect **critical incidents** whenever possible. Even a few critical incidents can be invaluable as examples or mini-cases, and they can be easily solicited in conjunction with questionnaires, individual interviews, or even group interviews.

   d. If normative or consensus data are needed on large numbers of scattered practitioners, use the **questionnaire** method. **Checklists** or **log diaries** can be included in the questionnaires if appropriate.

PROBLEM 7

What If The Future Role Does Not Currently Exist?

INTRODUCTION Sometimes an instructor thinks a performance analysis **cannot** be done because the role for which students are being prepared is a **new** position, and no competent practitioners currently exist.

However, a performance analysis can still be conducted under such circumstances. In fact, in some ways, it is even more important to verify an initial mastery description when the role is new and will affect existing health practitioners in new ways, than when the role is an established one. The materials in this section demonstrate some of the ways in which a performance analysis can be done in situations like this.

DIRECTORY

TYPE OF PROBLEM	RELATED ILLUSTRATION	SEE PAGE
No existing competent practitioners	7-A. A Model Advocate Dialogue: Simple Dental Procedures	B-57
New position being created	7-B. A Mini-Case: Practical Nutrition	B-60
Summary	Guidelines for Solving Problem 7	B-61

ILLUSTRATION 7-A

A MODEL ADVOCATE DIALOGUE: SIMPLE DENTAL PROCEDURES

INSTRUCTIONAL SITUATION

> Dr. Sanchez is a public health dentist who has been asked to teach medical assistants in Uruguay how to perform simple dental procedures. Although the position of medical assistant currently exists, these persons have never helped with dental problems, only with general medical problems.

Dr. Sanchez: How can I analyze **actual** professional performance for comparison with my initial mastery description when no competent practitioner currently exists? **No** medical assistants are performing these responsibilities now!

Model Advocate: Is there anyone around who *is* performing these or similar responsibilities?

Dr. Sanchez: Well sure, dentists here in the city do these things, but our medical assistants will be practicing in rural medical posts where they won't have nice offices or modern equipment. Only the basics. No one around here is doing exactly what these medical assistants will be doing.

Model Advocate: Could you observe what these urban dentists **are** doing and adapt their procedures as necessary, for example, when they use equipment you know will **not** be available to your medical assistants? After your observation you could interview them and ask how they **would** have done it if they hadn't had the particular instrument they were using.

Dr. Sanchez: Hmmm, I guess so. But wait a minute, you know I think there are a couple of traveling dentists who spend a week or so in one rural medical post and then move on to another. They carry around more equipment than our medical assistants will have, but at least they'd be familiar with the actual work conditions involved in these rural posts.

Model Advocate: They would certainly be better subject matter experts than urban dentists; but tell me, if these traveling dentists are already doing this type of dental work . . . why do you need to teach medical assistants to do it? And if your medical assistants are going to be putting these traveling dentists out of business, why would they be willing to cooperate with you?

Dr. Sanchez: Oh, our medical assistants won't be replacing these traveling dentists. There's plenty of dental work to be done; and as it now stands, villagers sometimes have to wait months before a traveling dentists arrives to pull a bad tooth or even to fill a cavity temporarily. We expect the traveling dentists to be delighted to have assistance with the simple jobs anyway, so they can concentrate on the more serious needs.

Model Advocate: I hope you're right; but if these traveling dentists have not yet been consulted on this project, they probably should be brought in as soon as

(Illustration 7-A, continued)

possible. Clearly they should have some say in defining this new role for the medical assistants and perhaps even in some of the teaching—they could be of immense help in giving feedback on field work.

Dr. Sanchez: Sure, why we might even have a kind of internship where a couple of medical assistants travel with a visiting dentist for a month or so. He could monitor their work on the simple procedures and they could assist him with the more complex work. Both would benefit.

Model Advocate: The prospects are exciting . . . but we're a bit ahead of ourselves. Right now we need to decide exactly how to determine to what extent your initial mastery description is representative of what the actual performance will be. If you can locate a couple of these traveling dentists, what method of performance analysis will you use?

Dr. Sanchez: I suppose I'll have to conduct individual interviews, since I doubt if I can find more than one in the same place at the same time.

Model Advocate: What about an observation interview? Your analyses of the skill components for these responsibilities are specific enough to serve as a checklist for observing actual performance, and you could supplement with questions about adapting the procedures.

Dr. Sanchez: Maybe I could arrange to accompany one of these traveling dentists for a day . . . but would that really be worth my time? I mean, he could just read over my mastery description here and tell me what he thinks, couldn't he?

Model Advocate: Sure, but it is amazing how much even an experienced practitioner learns when he observes another practitioner. Besides, you could get a feeling for the types of problems encountered, their relative proportions, and how the patients react to dental procedures. You might even see if you could do some work yourself under his supervision. There's nothing quite like the real experience for any teacher. I really do think it would be worth your making every effort to arrange such an experience for yourself.

Dr. Sanchez: Okay, I'll try . . . it might be kind of fun.

Model Advocate: Good! But what will you do if you can't locate one of these traveling dentists in time to arrange an observation? What about those urban dentists?

Dr. Sanchez: That's still a possibility I guess, but certainly wouldn't be as valuable. I think it would be even more helpful to have Dr. Ferronne look at my mastery description. He's actually in charge of this project; the whole thing was his idea. He's set up half of dozen of these medical posts himself and really knows their needs. Come to think of it, there's a couple of others right here in the city who've had experience in the rural areas. I'm sure I could arrange to interview them.

(Illustration 7-A, continued)

Model Advocate: You could save yourself time by getting them together in one room for a group interview.

Dr. Sanchez: That's true, and I'll bet they'll disagree on certain points too; so I could see how they resolve them.

Model Advocate: They'll also be more inclined to exchange stories, which will be excellent material for class examples later on. Could you include a dentist in these discussions to clarify any technical details.

Dr. Sanchez: I'm a dentist, but I suppose a second opinion would be helpful.

Model Advocate: If there is time for both the field experience with a traveling dentist and this group interview, the end result would be even better . . . but if you can only observe an urban dentist, this group interview is probably essential.

ILLUSTRATION 7-B

A MINI-CASE: PRACTICAL NUTRITION

INSTRUCTIONAL SITUATION	See Illustration 2-B, page B-14 for the instructional setting and examples of professional responsibilities for these volunteer health workers in an urban ghetto.

QUESTION 1

What types of individuals could be used as subject matter experts to help Dr. Myers determine if his initial mastery description is representative of what the volunteer health workers will actually be doing?

_ _

FEEDBACK

(a) Health workers performing similar functions in other similar low-income communities

(b) Local community leaders from the ghetto itself

(c) Individuals now working in community health centers where the volunteers will be located

(d) Health department officials involved in the decision to use volunteers for this purpose

---

QUESTION 2

What method(s) of performance analysis would you recommend to Dr. Myers, assuming that:

(a) he has limited time for a performance analysis,

(b) he has expertise in nutrition, not in ghetto life, and

(c) all the above types of individuals are available.

_ _

FEEDBACK

The best choice is probably a technical conference involving all four types of experts. Such a group can supply Dr. Myers with ample assistance in what to expect of his volunteers. In addition, the latter three groups listed above probably need to be brought into the planning phase for political reasons.

Another possible method of performance analysis for this case is the individual interview—preferably with health workers who are currently doing similar types of counseling, since they could share real-world experiences.

Critical incidents could be collected in conjunction with either of the above methods.

GUIDELINES FOR SOLVING PROBLEM 7

PROBLEM 7	How can one analyze actual professional performance if the future professional roles or responsibilities do not currently exist?

GUIDELINES

1. *For subject matter experts,*

   (a) try to locate substitute practitioners who are performing similar responsibilities under similar conditions,

   (b) use persons knowledgeable in the general subject area and/or in the professional situation of the future nonexistant role,

   (c) include individuals responsible for identifying the need for the new role and for sponsoring the course itself.

2. *For methods of performance analysis*, use the

   (a) *technical conference* (or group interview) when the new role involves a variety in inputs from different types of professionals and laymen,

   (b) *individual interview* (or questionnaire) when the experts cannot be collected for a common discussion, and

   (c) *observation interview* (with work participation) when a substitute health professional is available.

3. If appropriate, examine the reasons the new role is being established.

   - What problem(s) will the new role solve?
   - Is this the best way to solve these problems?

PROBLEM 8

How Does One Conduct
A Performance Analysis
and Revise the Mastery Description?

INTRODUCTION

Occasionally it is helpful to see the same example carried through several stages in the course design model. The illustration in this section has been designed to demonstrate the rationale, procedures, and conclusions of one instructor who conducted a performance analysis, located several performance discrepancies, and revised the initial mastery description on the basis of an analysis of the causes of these discrepancies.

This illustration also provides opportunity for you to practice identifying discrepancies, analyzing their causes, and suggesting changes.

DIRECTORY

TYPE OF PROBLEM	RELATED ILLUSTRATION	SEE PAGE
The basic procedure	8-A. An Extended Case: Biostatistics	B-63
Summary	No Guidelines for this section	

ILLUSTRATION 8-A

AN EXTENDED CASE: BIOSTATISTICS

INSTRUCTIONAL SITUATION

Dr. Mary Dromette is a biostatistics professor at Oakwood Dental School. The introductory biostatistics course has never been popular at Oakwood, and Dr. Dromette has decided to revise the course using the course design model described in Unit A. See Illustration 3-A, page B-17, for the initial list of professional responsibilities developed by Dr. Dromette for this course in Biostatistics. (**Note:** In this case, the component skills, knowledge, and attitudes were not analyzed until after the performance analysis had been completed and the initial list of responsibilities had been modified as explained below.)

THE PERFORMANCE ANALYSIS

The first step in analyzing the actual professional performance is to select and implement a method of performance analysis.

Method: The questionnaire method was selected, since it was thought desirable to collect information from a large number of practicing dentists to obtain consensus data on dentists' actual needs for and uses of biostatistics. Checklists were included within the questionnaire to facilitate recall.

Sample: All dentists attending the regional American Dental Association meetings in Springfield were asked to complete the questionnaire on registering. Only a handful of late arrivals failed to do so.

Materials: The questionnaire shown on pages B-64 and B-65 was designed and reproduced.

Results: 173 persons filled out the questionnaire.
      170 had been to dental school.
      152 were currently engaged in clinical practice.

More than 85% of those attending dental school recalled having taken a course in biostatistics. Almost 98% claimed to read research reports and of these, over half read between 5 and 10 articles per month. All the checklist steps in question 7 were performed by some respondents, although only 10% claimed to do all the steps all the time. Steps b, d, and f were the most frequently omitted. Over 80% of the population had **not** designed or conducted a research project since graduating from dental school. Of those who *had* conducted studies, over half had worked on more than 8 different studies. No additional responsibilities were uncovered by question 14.

(Illustration 8-A, continued)

QUESTIONNAIRE

The purpose of this investigation is to determine how useful biostatistics is to dentists in clinical practice. The results of this study will be used in designing a new biostatistics course at Oakwood School of Dentistry. Please read the questions carefully and follow the directions.

1. Are you engaged, at least part-time, in clinical dental practice?
   - ☐ Yes (Skip to question 3)
   - ☐ No (Go to question 2)

2. Did you attend dental school? ☐ Yes (Go on to question 3)
   ☐ No (Please answer no more questions and turn in your questionnaire)

3. Did you take biostatistics while in Dental School?
   - ☐ Yes
   - ☐ No (Go on to question 4)

4. Do you ever read professional dental journals and/or current research reports?
   - ☐ Yes (Go to question 5)
   - ☐ No (Skip to question 9)

5. Approximately how many different journal articles and reports do you read per month?

   (Go on to questions 6, 7 and 8)

6. Describe the source of the articles and reports you generally read?
   (i.e., specific journals, agencies, etc.) _____

   _____

7. Each item below is followed by a rating scale which is interpreted at the right. After each item, circle the appropriate number to indicate about how often you go through that step when you read articles or reports that describe the results of research.

SCALE INTERPRETATION:
0 = never
1 = about 25% of the time
2 = about 50% of the time
3 = about 75% of the time
4 = always

   a. Determine the purpose of the research being reported. 0 1 2 3 4

   b. Look for sources of bias in data collection procedures. 0 1 2 3 4

   c. Interpret data displayed in graphs, charts, or tables. 0 1 2 3 4

   d. Assess appropriateness of statistical procedures used. 0 1 2 3 4

   e. Interpret stated results of statistical tests. 0 1 2 3 4

   f. Obtain assistance from professional statistician if the reported statistics are beyond your understanding. 0 1 2 3 4

   g. Adopt dental procedures judged to be supported by adequate data. 0 1 2 3 4

8. Please explain your reasons for each rating of 0, 1, or 2 in question 7 above. (Use back of sheet if additional space is needed) _____

   _____

(Illustration 8-A, continued)

9. Have you ever designed and collected data for a research project of your own since you began clinical practice?

        ☐ Yes   (Skip to Question 11)
        ☐ No   (Go on to question 10)

10. Why have you never conducted such a study? Check all answers that apply; then skip to question 14.

        ☐ Not really interested
        ☐ Don't have time or resources
        ☐ Don't know how
        ☐ Other. Please specify:_____

_____

11. About how many times did you work on such a study, whether you completed it or not?_____(Go on to questions 12, 13, and 14)

12. Each of the items below is followed by a rating scale, interpreted at the right. After each item. Circle the appropriate number to indicate about how often you do the activity described when you work on research of your own.

SCALE INTERPRETATION:
0 = never
1 = about 25% of the time
2 = about 50% of the time
3 = about 75% of the time
4 = always

    a. Write out one or more hypotheses.   0 1 2 3 4

    b. Plan collection of data to minimize sources of bias.   0 1 2 3 4

    c. Plan data collection around the requirements of intended statistical tests.   0 1 2 3 4

    d. Display data in graphs, charts, or table.   0 1 2 3 4

    e. Calculate statistical significance.   0 1 2 3 4

    f. Write report on the results.   0 1 2 3 4

    g. Obtain assistance of a professional statistician.   0 1 2 3 4

13. Please explain your reasons for each rating of 0, 1, or 2 in question 12 above. (Use backside if needed)_____

_____

_____

14. Please describe below and on the backside of this sheet any *other* situations in which you use something you learned from your course on biostatistics. Explain what aspect of biostatistics you use and how. _____

_____

_____

_____

(THANK YOU. PLEASE TURN IN YOUR QUESTIONNAIRE.)

(Illustration 8-A, continued)

QUESTION 1	How did Dr. Dromette determine what tasks to include in the checklists for questions 7 and 12 of the preceding questionnaire?
	
	    a. From personal experience with these professional tasks
	    b. From her initial list of professional responsibilities
	    c. From a bibliographic search of tasks associated with biostatistics

FEEDBACK	The tasks were derived from the initial list of professional responsibilities that had been determined (somewhat arbitrarily) by Dr. Dromette during Task 1. In fact, the primary reason for developing the initial mastery description *before* analyzing actual performance is to have a basis for designing the verification study.
QUESTION 2	If you compare the checklist tasks (in questions 7 and 12) with the original professional responsibilities (page B-18), you will notice a number of differences in wording and, in some instances, sequencing or content. Why do you think the instructor changed the wording or meaning of these responsibilities when transferring them to the questionnaire?
FEEDBACK	The initial listing of professional responsibilities and the questionnaire have different purposes. The initial mastery description is a first approximation, a quick attempt to get something down in writing. The questionnaire, on the other hand, must be read and understood by a large number of individuals. It must be phrased in a style that can be quickly understood by the respondents.
IDENTIFYING DISCREPANCIES	After carrying out the performance analysis, Dr. Dromette's next step is to identify discrepancies between actual professional performance and the initial mastery description.
QUESTION 3	What performance discrepancies can you identify from the results described on pages B-63 and B-66?

FEEDBACK	Dr. Dromette identified the following two performance discrepancies:
	
	    (1) Very few practicing dentists collect data to test their own hypotheses.
	    (2) Most practicing dentists omit one or more steps when reading research articles. Steps b, d, and f were omitted more often than the others.

ANALYZING THE CAUSES OF DISCREPANCY 1	The first discrepancy listed above involves an entire category of responsibilities in the initial mastery description, that is, "when testing hypotheses of own choosing." Before revising the mastery description, Dr. Dromette's next step is to determine why practicing dentists rarely conduct research on their own. More specifically, is this discrepancy primarily the result of a skill/knowledge deficit, an attitude problem, and/or environmental factors?

(Illustration 8-A, continued)

The results from question 10 of the Questionnaire are pertinent to the above question. Here Dr. Dromette found that of those who had never conducted research,

59%	claimed they were "not really interested,"
83%	said they did not "have the time or resources,"
22%	admitted they "didn't know how," and finally
17%	specified as "other" reasons some variation of "not worth the effort."

QUESTION 4

Given the above data, to which of the following do you think this discrepancy can be primarily attributed?

  a. A lack of skills or knowledge.
  b. An inhibiting attitude.
  c. Inhibiting environmental factors.

FEEDBACK

The data seem to indicate that environmental factors (i.e., time and resources) are the primary causes of this discrepancy. However, Dr. Dromette suspected that attitude factors may be equally important. Not only do almost 60% admit they are not particularly interested in research, but an additional 17% took the time to explain that research was "not worth the effort." When she thought about this, Dr. Dromette realized there was very little payoff for a practicing dentist to conduct research; in fact, taking time for this type of activity was actually likely to be punishing (i.e., reduced income from patients).

REVISING THE MASTERY DESCRIPTION REGARDING DISCREPANCY 1

Having analyzed the causes of discrepancy 1, Dr. Dromette is ready to decide if and how she should revise her initial mastery description.

QUESTION 5

What would you recommend to Dr. Dromette regarding the revision of her mastery description to account for discrepancy 1?

FEEDBACK

Most people would agree that Dr. Dromette should simply discard the entire category of responsibilities related to "testing hypotheses" and focus (during this introductory course at least) on teaching her students to analyze the reported results of research. Students with research interests should be encouraged to take a more advanced course on experimental design.

(Illustration 8-A, continued)

DISCREPANCY 2 | The second discrepancy identified by Dr. Dromette was dentists who read reports of research studies rarely perform all the steps listed in the checklist. Most frequently omitted are:

Step b.   Looking for sources of bias in data collection procedures.
Step d.   Assessing the appropriateness of statistical procedures used.
Step f.   Obtaining the assistance of a professional statistician when the statistics are beyond their understanding.

When she examined the reasons given (in question 8) for omitting these steps, Dr. Dromette found:

(a) Most dentists do **not** feel competent to do steps b and d.
(b) Reasons for omitting step f include: (1) too much trouble, (2) not knowing any statisticians, (3) not thinking it worth the effort or time, and (4) not wanting to impose on someone.

QUESTION 6 | Given the above self-reported explanations, what do you think are the primary causes (i.e., skill/knowledge deficits, attitude problems, and/or environmental factors) for dentists failing to perform step b? step d? step f? What changes, if any, would you recommend Dr. Dromette make in her initial mastery description regarding each of these?

FEEDBACK | Skill/knowledge deficits appear to be the primary causes for the omission of steps b and d. Therefore, Dr. Dromette's course should probably emphasize these responsibilities. No change in the mastery description is indicated regarding steps b and d.

The primary cause for the omission of step f is probably a combination of attitudinal and environmental factors. Here Dr. Dromette decided to emphasize as knowledge components of this responsibility the advantages of obtaining advice from professional statisticians, ways to locate statisticians interested in dental research, and ways to maximize the use of a statistician's time (e.g., by inviting a statistician to local professional society meetings, etc).

(END OF CASE)

Chapter 5

IMPLEMENTATION PROBLEMS RELATED TO PHASE 2: DESCRIBING STUDENT COMPETENCIES

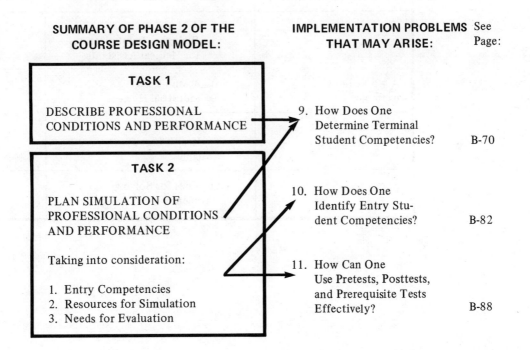

SUMMARY OF PHASE 2 OF THE COURSE DESIGN MODEL:	IMPLEMENTATION PROBLEMS THAT MAY ARISE:	See Page:
TASK 1 DESCRIBE PROFESSIONAL CONDITIONS AND PERFORMANCE	9. How Does One Determine Terminal Student Competencies?	B-70
TASK 2 PLAN SIMULATION OF PROFESSIONAL CONDITIONS AND PERFORMANCE Taking into consideration: 1. Entry Competencies 2. Resources for Simulation 3. Needs for Evaluation	10. How Does One Identify Entry Student Competencies?	B-82
	11. How Can One Use Pretests, Posttests, and Prerequisite Tests Effectively?	B-88

PROBLEM 9

How Does One Determine
Terminal Student Competencies?

INTRODUCTION At first it may appear easy to identify student competencies once the professional competencies have been described. However, sometimes it helps to:

(a) take a more careful look at the step-by-step process involved in actually determining terminal competencies,

(b) examine another worked-out example, and/or

(c) practice determining student competencies.

The materials in this section have been designed to provide for these needs.

DIRECTORY

TYPE OF PROBLEM	RELATED ILLUSTRATION	SEE PAGE
The basic process	9-A. A Model Advocate Dialogue: Immunization for Medical Assistants	B-71
A worked-out example	9-B. A Mini-Case: Industrial Hygiene	B-76
A chance to practice	9-C. A Mini-Case: Health Care Principles	B-79
Summary	Guidelines for Solving Problem 9	B-81

ILLUSTRATION 9-A

A MODEL ADVOCATE DIALOGUE:
IMMUNIZATION FOR MEDICAL ASSISTANTS

INSTRUCTIONAL SITUATION

See Illustration 5-B (pages B-42 to B-44) for relevant background on Dr. Josefs' course in immunization for medical assistants in Africa.

Entry Level: Students are in their third (and last) year of training before being assigned to work in health centers in villages or rural communities. They already have some background in related areas from previous courses in microbiology, infectious diseases, health services administration, etc. Specifically, they are familiar with the germ theory of disease, and with allergic reactions.

Resources for Simulation: The course is being given at an urban teaching hospital equipped with the usual supplies. About 15 students will take the course each time it is offered. The course extends 14 weeks, with one hour of lecture and two hours of lab each week. It is anticipated that part of the lab time will include supervised work in the hospital immunization clinic.

Needs for Evaluation: Each student must be assigned a final grade for the course, and Dr. Josefs expects to give a formal posttest at the end of the course. A pretest could provide useful information concerning what students already know, but Dr. Josefs does *not* think a prerequisite test would be useful.

Model Advocate: Now that you've established the professional performance of medical assistants, you are ready to determine what competencies your students should have when they complete your course. The first task here is to select those responsibilities from your revised mastery description for which you plan to design instruction. Do you plan to teach this first responsibility: "Identifies individuals in their areas who need immunization"?

Dr. Josefs: Oh yes, this is a very important responsibility.

Model Advocate: Okay, then we should describe the professional competency which is involved in this responsibility, by specifying the professional conditions and performance. What conditions will these medical assistants have available to them when they perform this first responsibility?

Dr. Josefs: Let's see. They will have the villages or rural communities where their health centers are located—and all the people who live there.

Model Advocate: And what performance is expected of them under these conditions?

Dr. Josefs: I thought I already described that in the skills column of my analyzed responsibility. (See page B-43.) They have to identify the target population, gain access to that target population, determine if immunization is needed by individuals, and so on.

(Illustration 9-A, continued)

Model Advocate: That's right. The performance to be described here is actually a **summary** of the skills that have already been analyzed. But since we are now ready to plan ways to **simulate** the professional situation during the course, it is useful to have the professional responsibility restated in terms of conditions and performance. This enables us to consider ways to simulate as many aspects of the professional situation as possible. Why don't we begin here by writing down these professional conditions and performance on a worksheet.

Dr. Josefs:

CONDITIONS	PERFORMANCE
Professional Competency: When given health centers where they will practice, and the villages or rural communities served by the respective health center . . .	. . . practitioners identify the target population, gain access to this population, and determine if immunization is needed by individuals in light of contraindications.

Model Advocate: Will it be possible to use this professional level as the **highest** level of simulation in your course?

Dr. Josefs: Oh no, that's impossible. These rural health centers are hundreds of miles from where this course will be taught.

Model Advocate: Okay, then what can you do to **simulate** these professional conditions and performance?

Dr. Josefs: Hmm . . . I could ask students to describe how they would go about identifying such individuals for immunization, assuming they had just arrived in the community where they will practice.

Model Advocate: Yes, you could do that. But is that really the best way to determine if your students are capable of carrying out this responsibility? Describing **how** one would do something is at the "talk about" level of simulation, and that's generally considered less preferable than a "doing" level of simulation. Isn't there some way to create conditions similar to those that will be encountered in their professional situations?

Dr. Josefs: Well I can't very well turn students loose in a new community to see if they can find everyone who needs to be immunized!

Model Advocate: No, but what about using case materials?

Dr. Josefs: Oh, I see what you mean . . . I can give them a description of some community similar to the ones they will enter, and have them determine the target populations, you know . . . which age groups would be at risk, such as infants, first graders, pregnant women, and so on.

(Illustration 9-A, continued)

Model Advocate: Sounds good! If it represents the highest level of simulation feasible for your course, why don't you add it to your worksheet.

Dr. Josefs:

CONDITIONS	PERFORMANCE
Professional Competency: When given the health centers where they will practice, and the villages or rural communities served by the respective health center . . .	. . . practitioners identify the target population, gain access to the target population, and determine if immunization is needed by individuals in light of contraindications.
Terminal Student Competency: When given a description of a particular community including indication of where babies are born, proportion of children in school, etc . . .	. . . students will determine the target populations, i.e., elegible age groups at high risk.

Model Advocate: Okay, now review what you've written. Is that sufficient to determine if students will be able to identify individuals for immunization in their own professional situation?

Dr. Josefs: Not really. A case like this only deals with **groups** and these students must also be able to determine if a given **individual** needs an immunization. Maybe I could use two separate terminal competencies for this one responsibility, and have students also work with real patients in the immunization clinic here at the hospital. They're supposed to spend some time in this clinic anyway as part of their lab experience for this course.

Model Advocate: I like the idea of using a two-part terminal competency, and it's great that students will have a chance to practice with real patients, but I wonder if clinic patients will be the best level of simulation for **evaluating** this responsibility. Will you be able to **measure** your students' success when they are working with real patients? Sounds as if it could take more of your time than it may be worth.

Dr. Josefs: Well, it would be too time-consuming for **me** to do, but their lab practice with patients will be supervised by Mrs. Karefa, the head nurse in our immunization clinic. She will be watching them very carefully anyway.

Model Advocate: Look, the way I see it, you have two problems here: **One**, you have no control over Mrs. Karefa. Can you rely on her judgments to be consistent from student to student? and **two**, the particular patients available for your

(Illustration 9-A, continued)

students on a given day (the day on which their evaluation is scheduled) may be atypical or too routine to be representative. Do you think this method of evaluation will give you a reliable estimate of student achievement?

Dr. Josefs: As far as Mrs. Karefa is concerned, she's very cooperative if not compulsive. If I develop some kind of rating scale or checklist for her to fill out for each patient a student works with, I'm sure she'll be consistent. You know, I'll bet Mrs. Karefa could even use these same evaluation sheets to give students feedback during their regular labs!

Model Advocate: That's an excellent idea. We'll consider it again when we get to Phase 3 and are ready to plan the checkpoints for the learning process. But now what about my second point? How representative would your test sample be?

Dr. Josefs: Well, if the evaluation sheets were used throughout the lab experience, and each student is in lab regularly, all should get their share of the different types of cases. But I see your point. Perhaps I shouldn't **judge** them during this learning process; and ensuring comparable patient loads for a fair evaluation **would** be difficult. Perhaps I could have students make decisions about case histories which I could design to sample the various situations that come up in the real world.

Model Advocate: That sounds good. Why don't you add it to your worksheet now.

Dr. Josefs:

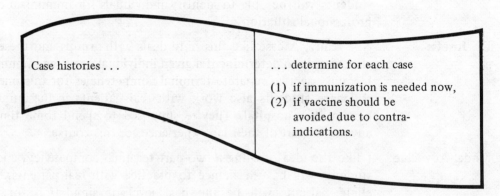

Case histories . . .

. . . determine for each case

(1) if immunization is needed now,
(2) if vaccine should be avoided due to contra-indications.

Model Advocate: That looks pretty good, but I wonder if the phrase "case histories" is specific enough to be helpful when you're ready to develop test items. For example, what data will you need for each of these case histories? And aren't there other resources that medical assistants have available to them when they perform this activity . . . , for instance, a copy of that immunization schedule?

Dr.Josefs: Oh, no—they have to know the immunization schedule by heart. It's really very simple! Besides, it would be much too awkward to be looking up this type of information once faced with a patient. But I could spell out these

(Illustration 9-A, continued)

case histories a bit more. Let's see, a case history should include the age, sex, general health, previous immunizations, perhaps some contraindications . . . but wait, that's not realistic—in the real world a complete medical history isn't simply handed to the medical assistant; he'll have to probe for much of this information. So my students have to know what to **ask** for . . . now I'm confused. What **should** my case histories include?

Model Advocate: Could you present **incomplete** cases and ask students to indicate first what additional information they would like to have and then discuss alternative decisions based on the information they received?

(Eventually this portion of the worksheet reads as follows:)

CONDITIONS	PERFORMANCE
(PROFESSIONAL COMPETENCY): When given the health centers where they will practice, and the villages or rural communities served by the respective health center . . .	. . . practitioners identify the target population, gain access to that population, and determine if immunization is needed by individuals in light of contraindications.
(TERMINAL STUDENT COMPETENCIES): (a) When given . . . description of a particular community including indication of where babies are born, percentage of children in school, etc. . . .	Students will . . . . . . determine the target populations, i.e., eligible age groups at high risk.
(b) case histories including age, sex, general health, and **incomplete** information related to previous immunizations and contraindications . . .	. . . determine for each case: (1) what additional information is necessary, and (2) what immunizations would be indicated depending on the nature of the additional data.

(END OF CASE)

ILLUSTRATION 9-B

A MINI-CASE: INDUSTRIAL HYGIENE

INSTRUCTIONAL SITUATION

Dr. King is teaching a course in industrial hygiene at a school of public health.

Entry Level: All students are MPH or MS candidates in environmental health sciences. Most already hold advanced degrees in medicine, engineering, social science, or some other related field. In addition, before taking this course in industrial hygiene, students will have taken courses in biostatistics, epidemiology, and human physiology.

Resources for Simulation: Labs equipped with environmental detection equipment are available at the school, and Dr. King has established good contact with local industrial firms so that field trips and site visits can be arranged. A total of 50 class hours has been allotted to the course, and this must include all labs and field trips. Course enrollment will be limited to 12 students.

Needs for Evaluation: Although the school does not require grades for all students (i.e., some elect to have only "pass" or "fail" appear on their grade transcripts), Dr. King plans to hold each student accountable for meeting certain criteria of performance. Thus he expects to have some form of posttest evaluation.

Purpose of the Course: To prepare students for the role of industrial hygienist, as related to the health and safety problems of workers in industrial and manufacturing settings.

Professional Responsibilities: An industrial hygienist . . .

1. Plans inspections of industrial settings.
2. Carries out inspections of industrial settings.
3. Identifies health and safety hazards in industrial settings.
4. Assigns priorities to hazards identified.
5. Recommends solutions to eliminate health and safety hazards.
6. Plans follow-up procedures to determine compliance with recommendations.

The skill/knowledge/attitude components of the third responsibility listed above are analyzed below.

(Illustration 9-B, continued)

Course Title: Industrial
Hygiene

ANALYZED RESPONSIBILITY

Responsibility No. 3: Identifies health and safety hazards in industrial settings.

A. Skills

1. Observes the workers, processes, equipment, products, and by-products.
2. Records observations as related to health and safety hazards.
3. Measures and records physical parameters: sound levels, dust, solvents, etc.
4. Analyzes medical and safety records of workers.
5. Recognizes health and safety hazards from above data.

B. Knowledge

1. Methods of observation and recording, including checklists, interview technique, audio- and videotape, diaries, and standard government forms.
2. Operation and calibration of environmental detection equipment.
3. Interpretation of environmental data.
4. Interpretation of medical and accident records.
5. Laws and regulations (a) governing the health and safety of industrial workers, and (b) defining the responsibilities and authority of inspectors.
6. Safety hazards by work type.
7. Health hazards: noise, dust, solvents, irritants, etc.
8. Implications of local political climate (the concerns and interactions of management, unions, and workers).

C. Attitudes

1. Physical and psychological well-being of industrial workers is more important than cost of controls.
2. Respect for the concerns of management, union leaders, and workers.
3. Importance of compromise and alternate solutions if immediate changes are not feasible.

(Illustration 9-B, continued)

CASE CONTINUED

The following worksheet illustrates the process Dr. King used to determine the highest feasible level of simulation for the terminal student competency.

Responsibility No. 3: Identifies health and safety hazards in industrial settings.

CONDITIONS	PERFORMANCE
(PROFESSIONAL COMPETENCY): When given access to a variety of industrial settings for individual observations, access to environmental detection equipment for a wide range of harmful agents and to medical records of workers . . .	. . . practitioners observe workers, record observations, measure physical parameters, analyze medical records, and identify with documentation the health and safety hazards of each setting.
(TERMINAL STUDENT COMPETENCY) When given access to a **particular** industrial setting for individual observation, access to a **limited** selection of detection equipment, and to medical records of workers . . .	. . . students will observe workers, record observations, measure physical parameters, indicate **what additional equipment is desirable**, analyze medical records, and identify with documentation the health and safety hazards of **particular** setting.
When given **a guided individual tour** of an industrial setting, access to limited detection equipment and to medical records of workers . . .	. . . students will observe workers, record observations, measure physical parameters, indicate what additional equipment is desirable, analyze medical records, and identify with documentation the health and safety hazards of particular setting. **Also, explaining what other workers or processes should have been observed.**
When given **a guided group tour of an** industrial setting with access to limited detection equipment and to medical records of the workers. . .	. . . same as above, except that total work will be shared by team of four students . . . each turning in a separate documented report with explanation of limitations due to constraints.

Not considered feasible for course. Could not get sufficient cooperation from local factories for each student to work individually

Highest level of simulation considered feasible for the course

ILLUSTRATION 9-C

A MINI-CASE: HEALTH CARE PRINCIPLES

INSTRUCTIONAL SITUATION

> See Illustration 4-A (page B-27) for background on this course for day-care directors, and page B-35 for the relevant analyzed responsibility as developed by Dr. Kakande.

QUESTION

What are the **conditions** and **performance** associated with the **professional competency** underlying this responsibility: "Identifies probable cases of protein calorie malnutrition (PCM) for referral to local health officers?"

FEEDBACK

Conditions: When given the children in the rural day-care centers which they will be directing

Performance: Practitioners observe children for clinical signs, measure arm circumference, take diet histories when appropriate, and decide whether or not to report each child as a probable case of PCM.

QUESTION

Since the various day-care centers are located in villages many miles from the course location, it would not be feasible to include the above activity as a terminal competency for the course. Below is a list of several successively lower levels of simulation. Which do you think is the **highest** level of simulation that would be feasible for Dr. Kakande to implement as a final evaluation for this course. Be sure to consider the instructional constraints: that is, a one-week government-sponsored course covering "all aspects of health care" which are relevant to a day-care director, and given at a modern city hospital with limited financial resources.

POSSIBLE LEVELS OF SIMULATION

1. When given a site visit to a local (urban) day-care center, students will identify children with probable cases of PCM.

2. When given a site visit to the emergency room of the city hospital, students will identify patients with probable cases of PCM.

3. Given color films or videotapes showing different children and their parents, some with PCM and some without, students will identify those children with probable cases of PCM for referral to the local health officer.

4. When given color slides of children with written diet and arm-circumference information on each case, students will identify those with probable cases of PCM for referral to the local health officer.

(Illustration 9-C, continued)

5. When given black-and-white photographs and written case information, students will identify probable cases of PCM for referral to the local health officer.

6. When given written cases (describing appearance of a child, arm circumference, and answers of parent to questions regarding the child's eating habits), students will identify probable cases of PCM for referral to the local health officer.

7. Students will describe the process they would use to identify a probable case of PCM for referral to the local health officer.

8. When given a list of clinical signs, some associated with PCM and others not, students will identify those signs which could indicate PCM.

_____

FEEDBACK

Dr. Kakande selected Level 4 as the highest level feasible within her course constraints. If more time were available, Levels 1 or 2 might be possible. However, even with the additional time, there is no guarantee that a local day-care center or the emergency room of a city hospital would have representative cases of protein calorie malnutrition on the day the site visit is arranged. Besides, the implementation of these simulation activities would be very difficult with a class as large as 20 students.

Level 3 (filmed or videotaped interviews) would be ideal in many respects; but even if the equipment were available, Dr. Kakande did not think she had the resources or expertise to locate sufficient numbers of malnourished and normal children and their parents, film appropriate interviews, edit the films and produce a final product in time for this course. Slides, on the other hand, can be borrowed or easily produced, and color slides are not significantly more expensive than black-and-white prints. Certainly color slides would be better than prints when it comes to showing clinical signs such as changes in hair color from black to reddish-brown.

GUIDELINES FOR SOLVING PROBLEM 9

PROBLEM 9   How does one determine terminal student competencies?

GUIDELINES

1. If it is not feasible to use the conditions and performance of the professional competency as the final level of simulation for students during the course, then back down from the conditions and performance of the professional level in small steps, considering the feasibility of each alternative before backing down another step.

2. Select as high a level of simulation as is feasible for **evaluating** terminal student competence. Be realistic about the:

   (a) **time** required to observe student performance, and
   (b) **need** for a representative and equivalent set of test stimuli for comparing the performance of all students fairly.

3. Remember that the "highest level of simulation" is selected for purposes of **evaluating** terminal student competencies. You can always use a still higher level of simulation for student practice during the course itself (e.g., have students practice with real patients, but evaluate them on the basis of a representative set of case studies).

PROBLEM 10

How Does One Identify Entry Student Competencies?

INTRODUCTION Entry student competencies are defined for two reasons:

(1) They are needed in Phase 3 when planning student learning; and
(2) They can serve as a set of specifications for a prerequisite test, just as terminal competencies serve as specifications for posttests (and pretests).

The problem here is just how to determine what the entry competencies are or should be for a given course.

The materials in this section demonstrate a recommended procedure for this process.

DIRECTORY

TYPE OF PROBLEM	RELATED ILLUSTRATION	SEE PAGE
Step-by-step demonstration of the procedure	10-A. An Extended Case: Health Care Principles	B-83
A worked-out example	10-B. A Mini-Case: Industrial Hygiene	B-86
Summary	Guidelines for Solving Problem 10	B-87

ILLUSTRATION 10-A

AN EXTENDED CASE: HEALTH CARE PRINCIPLES

INSTRUCTION SITUATION

See Illustration 4-A, page B-27, for background on this course for day-care center directors, and page B-35 for the relevant analyzed responsibility. Illustration 9-C, page B-79, is also related to this case.

To develop a list of specific entry competencies, it is necessary to examine each analyzed responsibility and determine what students, on entering the course, can reasonably be expected to know or do relative to each skill, knowledge, and attitude component.

QUESTION

Below is a portion of the analyzed responsibility for Dr. Kakande's course.

Identifies probable cases of protein calorie malnutrition (PCM) for referral to the local health officer.

SKILLS	KNOWLEDGE
1. **Observes children** for one or more clinical signs. Looks at: — general energy level — condition of arms, legs, belly, and face — color of the hair	(1) **Clinical signs of PCM:** a. marked weakness or inactivity b. skinny arms and legs c. pot belly (could also be worms) d. puffy eyes, face, arms, or legs e. hair color changes from black to reddish brown

Do you think Dr. Kakande's entering students (i.e., high school graduates coming directly from their native villages to take this course) will be able to recognize the clinical signs in children shown by color slides, assuming they have a list of what to observe?

FEEDBACK

Dr. Kakande thought her students would probably be able to recognize the signs when told to look for them, especially if normal children were available for comparison. Therefore, she wrote down as her first entry level competency the following:

When given . . .

Students will . . .

Children (some normal, some manifesting PCM); and a list of the clinical signs of PCM . . .

. . . recognize which clinical signs are exhibited by each child with PCM.

(Illustration 10-A, continued)

**CASE
CONTINUED**

Returning to the analyzed responsibility, the next skill and associated knowledge are as follows:

2. Measures arm circumference to determine if lower than standard:
 	
   a. Has child bend arm at elbow, etc.
	(2) How arm circumference test works:
	
	   – upper arm is made of a bone wrapped in muscle and skin, etc.

Dr. Kakande decided that her students would probably already be familiar with tape measures and know how to use one. Most of her students will have taken sewing, math, or some science course in high school during which measurement was taught.

Dr. Kakande wrote out the following entry competency:

When given . . .

Students will . . .

A tape measure and a cylinder . . .

. . . measure the circumference of the cylinder.

In the same way as above, Dr. Kakande methodically examined each skill, knowledge, and attitude component to determine what previous experiences may have prepared students for learning this responsibility. The material below shows the questions Dr. Kakande asked herself, the answers she gave, and the entry competencies she developed when appropriate.

(Illustration 10-A, continued)

QUESTIONS DR. KAKANDE ASKED HERSELF:	ANSWERS:	ENTRY STUDENT COMPETENCIES
Have my students had any previous experience in interviewing or taking dietary histories?	Probably *not*. Of course they have asked isolated questions, but probably will *not* know how to probe for specific information.	
Are the concepts **protein** and **calorie** new to my students?	No, in high school they studied protein, carbohydrates, vitamins, etc. They may also have learned common sources of each.	When given a list of nutritional elements (e.g., protein, vitamin, etc.), a list of nutritional functions, and a list of common sources of each element . . . students will match each nutritional element to its respective function and source.
Are students familiar with the types of foods commonly eaten in their villages?	Yes; they should know the staple foods in their own villages, but probably do *not* know the nutritional content of these foods.	When given directions, students will list the most common foods eaten in their own villages.
What in their backgrounds might have prepared students for deciding whether to refer a given child to the local health officer?	They may know the health officer exists, and common sense would lead them to seek help for any seriously ill or injured child; but they won't know the criteria for diagnosing cases of PCM.	When asked what they would do with a seriously ill or injured child, students will indicate referral to the local health officer as an option.
Are they aware of the prevalence of PCM and of the consequences of failing to treat it?	Probably **not**.	
Will they know how to handle a child gently so as not to alarm him/her?	Probably. Most girls growing up in a village get plenty of practice with younger siblings.	
Will they know how to ask questions in a casual nonthreatening way?	Perhaps some will; others will not.	

(END OF CASE)

ILLUSTRATION 10-B

A MINI-CASE: INDUSTRIAL HYGIENE

INSTRUCTIONAL SITUATION

See Illustration 9-B beginning on page B-76 for background on this case.

WORKED-OUT ENTRY LEVEL COMPETENCIES

Dr. King developed the following list of entry student competencies for his third responsibility.

Course Title: Industrial Hygiene

ENTRY COMPETENCIES

Responsibility No. 3: Identifies health and safety hazards in industrial settings.

CONDITIONS	PERFORMANCE
When given . . .	Students will . . .
a. A list of harmful industrial agents . . .	. . . identify body systems affected (80% accuracy).
b. A list of terms (such as calibrate, toxic, etc. . . .	. . . define correctly 75% of the terms.
c. A set of lung X-rays, some diseased, some not . . .	. . . identify diseased lungs (at rate of 1 X-ray/min).
d. Checklists for observing three sets of simple procedures . . .	. . . use the checklists while observing videotapes of the procedures being performed (in three different settings).

GUIDELINES FOR SOLVING PROBLEM 10

PROBLEM 10 How does one identify and describe entry student competencies?

GUIDELINES 1. For each analyzed responsibility, examine each skill/knowledge, and attitude component in terms of your students' general backgrounds. Ask yourself:

- How much background will my students have had in relation to this component before entering this course?

- Have these students ever taken a course in which some aspect of this material would have been covered?

- Have they had experience with this component in any way?

- Are there any specific prerequisites that can reasonably be expected of these students?

2. Convert each identified entry level knowledge and skill into a competency by specifying conditions and performance.

3. Do not include entry competencies known to be common to only a small proportion of the students.

PROBLEM 11

How Can One Use Pretests, Posttests, and Prerequisite Tests Effectively?

INTRODUCTION Many instructors think they are finished once they have scored tests and assigned grades. They do not bother to analyze the performance of the class as a whole. This may be because they do not realize how much can be learned by examining:

(a) a distribution of the scores from the entire class,
(b) a pair of pretest-posttest score distributions, or
(c) patterns of student errors.

By displaying performance data from a group of students in particular configurations, one can learn a great deal about those students, the effectiveness of the instruction, and the quality of the evaluation instrument.

The materials in this section have been designed to teach you how to examine and interpret performance data so that you will be able to use the results of pretests, posttests, and prerequisite tests more effectively.

DIRECTORY

TYPE OF PROBLEM	RELATED ILLUSTRATION	SEE PAGE
What can be learned from a distribution of class scores?	11-A. A Feedback Exercise: Interpreting a Score Distribution	B-89
What can be learned from a pair of pretest-posttest score distributions?	11-B. A Feedback Exercise: Determining the Influence of Instruction	B-91
What can be learned from examining patterns of student errors?	11-C. A Feedback Exercise: Analyzing an Error Matrix	B-93
Summary	Guidelines for Solving Problem 11	B-97

ILLUSTRATION 11-A

A FEEDBACK EXERCISE: INTERPRETING A SCORE DISTRIBUTION

INTRODUCTION Below are displayed six possible score distributions. Scores are plotted on the horizontal axis on an arbitrary scale of 100. The frequency with which each score occurs is plotted on the vertical axis. For example, on distribution 3, the most frequent score is 50. Assume 500 students were tested so that the distributions represent "idealized" results.

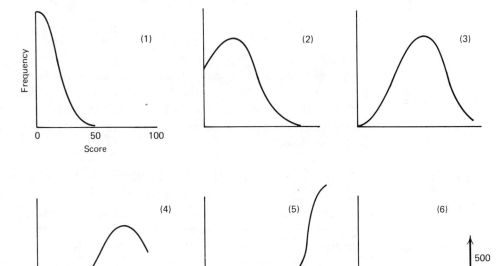

QUESTION 1 Which distribution represents the best posttest performance attainable under realistic instructional conditions?

FEEDBACK # 5, which has a high mean score with relatively few low scores. Some people choose the symmetrical or "normal" curve (# 3) as most desirable, because such a distribution discriminates among different levels of student attainment. However, when one wants all students to achieve the terminal competencies, the theoretically ideal distribution is a straight vertical line at score 100 (as in # 6), indicating all students got all items correct. Distribution # 5 is a good approximation of this ideal and is probably the best attainable under realistic conditions.

QUESTION 2 On the basis of your own experience as a student and teacher, which distribution represents the "most typical" posttest results?

(Illustration 11-A, continued)

FEEDBACK

In the learning of traditional "academic" content, it is fairly typical to have an average final examination score of about 75%, best represented by distribution 4. However, distribution 3 may very well be typical in some cases where students of varied backgrounds are taught a variety of content, or where standards of evaluation are much higher than standards of teaching.

QUESTION 3

Which distribution represents adequate or "passing" student performance?

FEEDBACK

There is no simple answer to this question despite its importance to most evaluation efforts. For example, in the training of surgeons or commercial aircraft pilots, it is crucial that all students perform certain tasks nearly perfectly all the time. Distribution 6 would be ideal in these cases, but 5 may be more typical. However, on any distribution one can select a cutoff score that must be met by any student who is to pass. Note that a cutoff score as low as 75% on distribution 3 would fail most of the students and suggest that the instruction was inadequate. Explicit pass-fail and/or grading decisions must be made by all teachers, and it is important to do so on a rational basis.

QUESTION 4

If one were to administer a **pretest** to an unselected group of individuals who had received varying amounts of opportunity to learn the subject matter being tested, which distribution would probably result?

FEEDBACK

Distribution 3 can be expected to result from the operation of random processes. However, administering a pretest to a group preselected to be more or less likely to know the subject matter will skew the curve.

QUESTION 5

If the skills and knowledge measured on a **prerequisite** test have been taught at some time during students' background, which distribution is likely to result?

FEEDBACK

Distribution 4. The past instruction will have moved the distribution up from a normal curve with a mean of 50. It is unlikely, however, that one ever finds prerequisite test results similar to distribution 5. Such a curve is too systematically high for scores from a variety of individuals who will have been taught under a variety of circumstances at varying times in the past.

ILLUSTRATION 11-B

A FEEDBACK EXERCISE: DETERMINING THE INFLUENCE OF INSTRUCTION

INTRODUCTION In each **pair** of score distributions below, one curve corresponds to the pretest data and the other to posttest data for the same unit of instruction. The **change** in score distributions between pre- and posttest is referred to as the "gain."

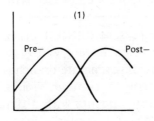
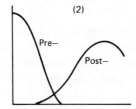
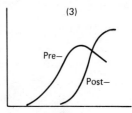

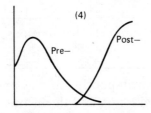
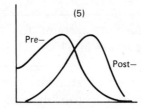
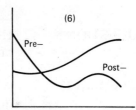

QUESTION 1 Which pair(s) of pre-posttest distributions show(s) the **most** gain?

FEEDBACK Distributions 2 and 4 seem by inspection to show approximately equal gains. Distribution 6 also shows considerable gain, but because of the bimodal nature of the curves, it is difficult to compare this gain to that of the other curves.

QUESTION 2 Which pair(s) of distribution show the **least** pre- posttest gains?

FEEDBACK Distributions 3 and 5, which by inspection seem to show approximately equal gains.

QUESTION 3 If one is interested in high-quality **student** performance at the end of instruction, which pair of distributions is preferable: 2 or 3?

(Illustration 11-B, continued)

FEEDBACK | Distribution 3 because posttest results are higher than in distribution 2. If hiring practitioners on the basis of test results, one would prefer to draw from the pool of individuals represented in 3 rather than in 2, even though the individuals in 2 showed more gain between pre- and posttest.

QUESTION 4 | Which distribution, those in 2 or in 3, indicate the greater need for branching (i.e. for creating separate instructional tracks for students on the basis of their pretest performance)? How about 4 compared with 5?

FEEDBACK | The distributions in 3 and 5 represent difficult instructional situations in which the students' entry competencies are widely scattered, resulting in small post-instruction gains. Providing separate branches for those with more or less preknowledge of the course content would have provided the individualized attention needed by students with different levels of entering competencies. In distributions 2 and 4, students appear to know less when they enter the instruction, but gain more. Here branching probably is **not** indicated.

QUESTION 5 | How do you account for the bimodal distributions of the pretest and posttest scores in 6?

FEEDBACK | Although most students performed poorly on the pretest, a number did quite well and probably could have bypassed the instruction. Posttest results were not consistent, because of poor teaching and/or wide variation in the entry level characteristics of the students. Deficits in assumed prerequisites or in general ability could have prevented some students from learning, as could the nature and quality of the instruction.

ILLUSTRATION 11-C

A FEEDBACK EXERCISE: ANALYZING AN ERROR MATRIX

INTRODUCTION The overall results of the pre- and posttests for a unit of instruction are displayed in the score distributions below, with each bar of the histogram representing all scores within a five-point interval. These data are displayed in essentially the same manner as the idealized group data from the previous two exercises; however, here only 10 students were involved instead of 500.

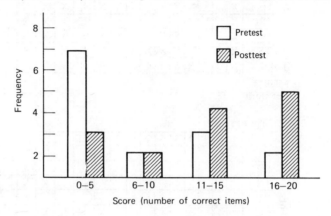

QUESTION 1 To which pair of idealized curves on page B-91 do the above distributions most closely correspond?

FEEDBACK NO. 6

INTRODUCTION CONTINUED Below, the same data as shown above are presented in a pair of student-by-item error matrices. These more detailed displays permit one to analyze the possible "causes" of the overall results observed in the group data, that is, to diagnose problems with individual items and with individual students.

Before proceeding with an analysis of these matrices, a few basic points about the display must be explained:

(a) The pre- and posttests are the **same** test used both before and after instruction.
(b) Each of the 10 students, KL to TS, took both tests.
(c) Each number along the top of the matrix represents a separate test item.
(d) An "X" indicates a student error. Errors are totaled in each column, and total items **correct** (blank cells) are totaled in each row.

(Illustration 11-C, continued)

PRETEST	1	2	3	4	5	6	7	8	9	10	11	12	13	14	15	16	17	18	19	20	Total Score	Percent Correct
KL														X			X				18	90
DP	X		X	X		X	X	X	X	X	X	X	X	X	X	X	X			X	4	20
TR	X		X			X	X		X		X	X	X				X		X	X	9	45
RR	X		X	X	X	X	X	X	X	X	X	X	X	X	X	X	X		X	X	2	10
CE	X		X	X		X	X	X	X	X	X	X	X	X	X	X	X		X	X	3	15
JC							X	X	X	X	X	X		X							13	65
HST	X		X	X	X		X	X	X	X	X	X	X	X		X	X		X	X	4	20
JBC	X		X					X	X	X	X			X							12	60
DOM	X		X	X	X	X	X	X	X		X	X	X	X	X	X	X	X	X	X	1	5
TS	X		X	X	X	X	X	X	X		X	X	X	X	X	X	X	X	X	X	1	5
Total errors per item	8	0	7	8	6	4	6	8	7	9	8	9	9	10	5	6	8	2	6	7		

POSTTEST	1	2	3	4	5	6	7	8	9	10	11	12	13	14	15	16	17	18	19	20	Total Score	Percent Correct
KL																		X			19	95
DP													X					X			18	90
TR													X	X				X			17	85
RR				X										X				X			17	85
CE										X	X	X	X	X				X			14	70
JC				X						X	X	X	X	X				X			13	65
HST								X		X	X	X	X	X				X			13	65
JBC	X		X	X	X	X	X						X	X	X	X	X	X		X	6	30
DOM	X		X	X		X	X			X	X	X	X		X	X	X	X	X		4	20
TS	X		X	X		X	X	X		X	X	X	X	X			X	X	X	X	4	20
Total errors per item	3	0	3	4	3	2	4	3	0	5	5	5	7	9	2	2	3	10	2	3		

Item Diagnosis

QUESTION 1

Which items show essentially no gain, or even a loss, from pretest to posttest?

FEEDBACK

Items 2, 14, 18, and maybe 13. Item 2 shows no errors on either test; item 14 shows a gain of only one; item 13 shows a marginal gain of 2; and item 18 goes from 2 errors on the pretest to 10 on the posttest.

QUESTION 2

Give possible explanations for these results, item by item.

(Illustration 11-C, continued)

FEEDBACK

Item 2: Students already knew the material to be taught, or the question was worded in a manner to give away the answer.

Items 13 and 14: May be due to inadequate instruction, or to poor items, for example, ambiguous, tricky, etc.

Item 18: The students may have been taught something incorrect, which led to errors; a scoring error may have been made on the posttest; or there may be a typographical error in the posttest or its answer key.

Student Diagnosis

QUESTION 3

Most of the students showed a gain from pretest to posttest. Did any students show **no gain** or even a **loss** from pretest to posttest?

FEEDBACK

A loss of six was demonstrated by JBC but JC had the same number correct (13) on both pretest and posttest.

QUESTION 4

On the basis of posttest scores, which students did not show adequate mastery of what was taught?

FEEDBACK

JBG, DOM, and TS; and depending on the standards applied, perhaps CE, JC, and HST (60 to 70% is usually considered a borderline score).

QUESTION 5

Which students did not **need** the instruction in the first place?

FEEDBACK

KL, with a pretest score of 18; and maybe JC, who made a pretest score of 13.

QUESTION 6

What about the bizarre performance of JBC? What are some possible explanations for his doing more poorly on the posttest than on the pretest?

FEEDBACK

(a) Student error in marking answer sheet, for example, by putting all answers off by one space on the answer sheet.

(b) Physical illness while taking the posttest.

(c) Poor motivation or deliberate attempt to distort the test results.

(d) Mistake in scoring, and so on.

A suitable solution to this problem must remain hypothetical until further evidence is gathered.

(Illustration 11-C, continued)

CONCLUDING COMMENT

The above type of analysis could continue further with the present set of data, and would be repeated after the next, revised administration of the unit of instruction. However, an important aspect of this type of analysis has not been dealt with here. This concerns interpretation of specific errors made, and how one revises instruction and test items on the basis of such an analysis. This type of analysis requires access to the instruction itself, the actual test items, and how many students make what types of errors on each test item.

GUIDELINES FOR SOLVING PROBLEM 11

PROBLEM 11   How can one use pretest, posttests, and prerequisites tests effectively? That is, how can one analyze the performance data from an entire class to determine the effectiveness of the instruction, the quality of the testing instrument, and the nature of individual student problems?

GUIDELINES

1. Prepare a frequency distribution or histogram of the final scores for every test you administer. Determine the quality of overall student performance by examining how the scores are skewed.

2. If pretest data is available for the same test instrument as posttest data, include both distributions on the same graph to determine how much the overall performance was improved by the instruction.

3. For **item diagnosis** when only the posttest data are available, prepare a student-by-item error matrix and look for items that were:

   (a) missed by **high** scoring students   →   may indicate unsuccessful teaching or a poor item

   (b) passed by **low** scoring students   →   may be too easy or a "giveaway" item

When both pretest and posttest data are available for the same test instrument, look for items that have:

   (a) **high errors** on pretest; **low errors** on posttest   →   probably a "good" item: shows desired change after instruction

   (b) **low errors** on pretest; **high errors** on posttest   →   either item is ambiguous to one who knows something about the subject, or else the instruction was misleading

   (c) **high errors** on both pre- and posttest   →   could indicate unsuccessful teaching or poor item (i.e., ambiguous, off-target behavior, etc.)

   (d) **low errors** on both pre- and posttest   →   probably too easy or a "giveaway" item (i.e., should not have been included in course or bypassing should be provided)

4. For **student diagnosis**, examine the error patterns of each student with a high error rate. If items were missed that better students passed, try to infer why they were missed by examining the actual items and the responses given.

   • Did the student lack some prerequisite skill?

   • Did the student fail to understand a particular recurring concept?

   • Did the student fail to learn across-the-board?

Chapter 6

IMPLEMENTATION PROBLEMS RELATED TO PHASE 3: PLANNING STUDENT LEARNING

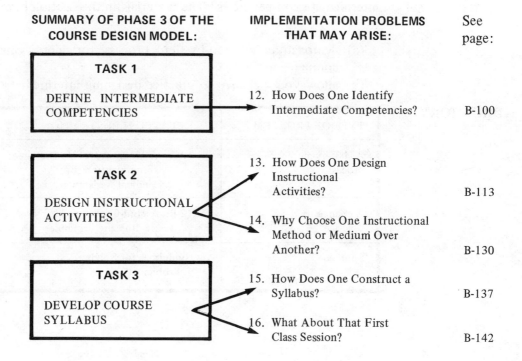

SUMMARY OF PHASE 3 OF THE COURSE DESIGN MODEL:	IMPLEMENTATION PROBLEMS THAT MAY ARISE:	See page:
TASK 1 DEFINE INTERMEDIATE COMPETENCIES	12. How Does One Identify Intermediate Competencies?	B-100
TASK 2 DESIGN INSTRUCTIONAL ACTIVITIES	13. How Does One Design Instructional Activities?	B-113
	14. Why Choose One Instructional Method or Medium Over Another?	B-130
TASK 3 DEVELOP COURSE SYLLABUS	15. How Does One Construct a Syllabus?	B-137
	16. What About That First Class Session?	B-142

PROBLEM 12

How Does One Identify Intermediate Competencies?

INTRODUCTION   A comprehensive and well-designed set of intermediate competencies is probably the best way to assure that students will be actively involved in their learning process.

But just how does one develop a comprehensive, well-designed set of intermediate competencies? The materials in this section have been designed to:

(a) demonstrate a step-by-step process for identifying intermediate competencies,
(b) allow you a chance to practice designing intermediate competencies.

DIRECTORY

TYPE OF PROBLEM	RELATED ILLUSTRATION	SEE PAGE
A step-by-step process	12-A. A Model Advocate Dialogue: Immunization for Medical Assistants	B-101
A chance to practice	12-B. A Mini-Case: Health Care Principles	B-107
Summary	Guidelines for Solving Problem 12	B-112

ILLUSTRATION 12-A

A MODEL ADVOCATE DIALOGUE:
IMMUNIZATION FOR MEDICAL ASSISTANTS

INSTRUCTIONAL SITUATION

See Illustrations 5-B (page B-42) and 9-A (page B-71) for background on this case, analyzed responsibilities, and terminal student competencies.

Model Advocate: Developing *intermediate competencies* involves continuing from where you stopped when identifying terminal competencies, only now you need to identify still lower levels of simulation through which students should progress on their way to the highest level of simulation identified for the entire responsibility. Can you think of any ways to evaluate student learning **before** having them determine the target population for a hypothetical community or work on your incomplete individual case histories?

Dr. Josefs: Not for identifying target populations—that's really very easy. But perhaps before giving students incomplete case histories, I should give them a series of **complete** cases for which to decide appropriate immunizations. Would that represent an intermediate competency?

Model Advocate: Certainly. It represents an approximation of real-world performance but does not simulate the professional level as closely as the incomplete case histories do. And one must be able to make decisions when presented with all the relevant data before being ready to determine what data are missing from a given case. Do you think you will need any still lower levels of simulation regarding this entire responsibility?

Dr. Josefs: I don't think we need any more **lower** levels of simulation, but shouldn't we include here practice with patients in the lab? Earlier we decided not to use lab practice as the highest level of simulation for evaluating the **terminal** competence of students, but I do want students to have this practice and receive feedback from Mrs. Karafa.

Model Advocate: Good point. Let's include the lab practice as an intermediate level of simulation regarding the entire responsibility. Actually, though, this should be the first intermediate competency, since it's a higher level of simulation than the case studies. Now, are we ready to start identifying competencies for isolated components of this responsibility.

Dr. Josefs: I don't think we need to bother with the components. After all, it looks like students will be getting plenty of practice both with case studies and with live patients. They'll have to learn all the skill, knowledge, and attitude components to be able to work on these intermediate competencies regarding the entire responsibility.

(Illustration 12-A, continued)

Model Advocate: Ah, but what if they **fail** to perform adequately on the case histories? Would you know **why** they failed? In other words, say a student makes the wrong decision about needed immunizations for a particular case, would you know if he was confused about the immunization schedule, didn't remember some important contraindication, or simply failed to read through the case carefully enough? If not, how could you give that student remedial help or improve your own instruction next time you give the course?

Dr. Josefs: You mean I have to ask my students to reproduce each little bit of information and perform every tiny step of the procedure in isolation before letting them put it all together, just so I can diagnose the cause of some hypothetical failure?

Model Advocate: Not at all. That's why it's so important to **select** these intermediate competencies carefully. Only design competencies for those components of the analyzed responsibility that are either *omitted from* or *prerequisite to* successful performance on the terminal competency and/or intermediate competencies for the entire responsibility. For example, before your students can handle the case histories or patients, they must know the immunization schedule. Wouldn't you like to have a mechanism to assess student mastery of this schedule **before** you present them with your case histories?

Dr. Josefs: Yes, I guess that would be a good idea. Perhaps I can have them reconstruct the immunization schedule from memory. So that's my first "component" competency, huh? Let me write that down . . . *(pause)* . . . Hey! I have a "performance" here but what are my "conditions?" I'm not going to "give" my students anything—they have to recall the schedule from memory!

Model Advocate: What will serve as the test stimulus? **When** . . . under what conditions . . . will students reproduce the schedule?

Dr. Josefs: When I tell them to!

Model Advocate: Then your **telling** them **is** the test stimulus. Simply write "test item" or "directions" in the "conditions" column. This is to remind you, when you are ready to construct test items, that you must take some time to **phrase** your directions to the students.

(Illustration 12-A, continued)

Dr. Josefs:

Course Title: Immunization for
Medical Assistants

INTERMEDIATE COMPETENCIES

Responsibility: Identifies individuals from their areas who need immunization.

CONDITIONS	PERFORMANCE
When given . . .	Students will . . .
(Regarding Entire Responsibility:)	
1. Patients in hospital immunization clinic . . .	. . . decide what vaccine is needed and, if contraindicated, what to do.
2. Complete case histories . . .	. . . decide what immunizations are needed, and if contraindicated, what to do.
(Regarding Isolated Components:)	
3. Directions . . .	. . . reconstruct from memory the complete immunization schedule.

Model Advocate: That's fine. But the best way to develop intermediate competencies for components is to systematically examine each item listed in the analysis of the responsibility. After all, you already specified everything you think someone must be able to do or know to execute this responsibility. The immunization schedule is listed as the third knowledge component in your analysis of this responsibility. What about the first component in your skills column?

> 1. Identifies target population:
>
>   a. Determines eligible ages.
>   b. Identifies high-risk groups.

Dr. Josefs: That component is already being handled by any first terminal competency. However, to do this, students must know the meaning of "target population" and "high-risk group."

Model Advocate: How will you find out if they know what these terms mean?

Dr. Josefs: I could ask them for definitions.

(Illustration 12-A, continued)

Model Advocate: Will simple definitions be sufficient to demonstrate understanding of these terms? Some definitions can be memorized without comprehension. Often it is better to ask for an example of a term, or for both a definition and an example. Recognition of examples is actually closer to the real-world use of most terms.

Dr. Josefs: I think a simple definition of "target population" will be sufficient, but perhaps I should ask for an example of a "high-risk group" in addition to the definitions.

Model Advocate: Fine. Now what about skill no. 2 and its corresponding knowledge component?

2. Gains access to target pop.: a. Contacts community institutions. b. Gives health education talks. c. Screens clients coming to health centers.	What a community needs to know about immunization.

Dr. Josefs: That step was so large that I developed and analyzed a separate responsibility for it (*See Illustration* 5-B, page B-42).

Model Advocate: Then you'll decide how to evaluate it when you work on that responsibility. What about skill no. 3?

3. Determines if immunization is needed by individuals: a. Determines age.   b. Checks for previous immunizations (scars, etc).   c. Recalls immunization schedule to decide if immunization is needed.

Dr. Josefs: I see no reason to test for this behavior apart from the case histories. If they know the immunization schedule by heart, then this step is fairly straightforward. In fact, the same is true for skill 4, "consider contraindications." However, I must be certain they know the contraindications before they try any of the intermediate levels of simulation for the overall responsibility.

Model Advocate: How will you determine whether or not your students know these contraindications?

Dr. Josefs: I could give them a list of the vaccines and have them describe the contraindications for each. In the real world they must recall these from memory each time they consider giving a specific vaccine.

(Illustration 12-A, continued)

Model Advocate: Now, the only component left in your knowledge column is the background theory. Do you need to check student progress on this background knowledge?

> *Background Theory:*
>
> — Responses of an organism to an infectious agent.
> — Ways to protect organism
>   a. isolation.
>   b. passive or active immunization.

Dr. Josefs: Oh, yes—I want to be sure they understand what's involved here. I can have them list the responses of an organism to an infectious agent and list the ways an organism can be protected.

Model Advocate: That's one way; but is it really important for your students to **recall** this information? Will they go around listing these things in the real world?

Dr. Josefs: Hmmm . . . no, I guess not. These concepts should serve as a kind of frame of reference; you know, as a model for what is going on with infections and immunization.

Model Advocate: Could you find out if they've acquired this frame of reference without having them list it?

Dr. Josefs: Perhaps I could construct some multiple-choice items which would require understanding but permit recognition instead of asking for total recall.

Model Advocate: Good idea! Now that you've considered each skill and knowledge component you may be finished. But it's a good idea to review your attitude column, too, because sometimes important content elements show up as attitudes. What do you think? Is there anything here which needs progress checking?

> — Understands the importance of immunization for a community.
> — Appreciates the value of having and using an immunization schedule.
> — Realizes the seriousness of these contraindications if not discovered.

Dr. Josefs: Yes, I think I'd like to know if my students understand the advantages of using an immunization schedule. I can probably add one or two multiple-choice questions on that too.

(Illustration 12-A, continued)

INTERMEDIATE COMPETENCIES

Responsibility: Identifies individuals from their area who need immunization.

CONDITIONS	PERFORMANCE
When given . . .	Students will . . .
(Regarding Entire Responsibility:)	
1. Patients at hospital immunization clinic . . .	. . . decide what vaccine is needed and if contraindicated, what to do.
2. Complete case histories	. . . decide what immunizations are needed, and if contraindicated, what to do.
(Regarding Isolated Components:)	
3. Directions . . .	. . . reconstruct from memory the complete immunization schedule.
4. The terms "target population" and "high-risk group" . . .	. . . define both terms and give an example of a high-risk group.
5. List of vaccines . . .	. . . describe: (a) nature of contraindications for each vaccine, and (b) how to deal with each.
6. Multiple-choice items . . .	. . . recognize: (a) types of responses to infectious agents, (b) ways organism can be protected, and (c) advantages of using an immunization schedule.

ILLUSTRATION 12-B

A MINI-CASE: HEALTH CARE PRINCIPLES

INSTRUCTIONAL SITUATION

See Illustration 4-A (page B-27) for background on this course for day-care center directors. Illustrations 9-C (page B-79) and 10-A (page B-83) are related to this same case.

In working on this case, you may need to refer to the following:

Analyzed Responsibility — Page B-109
Professional, Terminal and Entry Competencies — Page B-110

QUESTION

A worksheet for developing Intermediate Competencies for this responsibility has been begun on page B-108.

Complete this worksheet by designing competencies for isolated skill, knowledge, and attitude components of this responsibility. Examine each item in the analysis on page B-109, and ask yourself:

- Is this component covered adequately by one or more of the intermediate competencies regarding the entire responsibility? If not, should this component be covered by a separate checkpoint?

- Is it necessary that students know or can do this before they will be able to perform the overall responsibility? If so, should this component be checked in isolation before being combined with others?

- If students fail at a higher level of simulation, could this component be responsible? If so, would a separate intermediate competency enable me to find out that this component was the problem?

After deciding which components should be covered by intermediate competencies, develop specifications for progress tests by describing conditions and performance, as modeled in the previous illustration.

FEEDBACK

The intermediate competencies identified by Dr. Kakande are shown on page B-111.

(Illustration 12-B, continued)

<table>
<tr><td colspan="2" style="text-align:right;"><u>Course Title:</u> Health Care Principles
for Day-Care Directors</td></tr>
<tr><td colspan="2" style="text-align:center;">INTERMEDIATE COMPETENCIES
<u>Responsibility:</u> Identifies probable cases of PCM for referral to local health officers.</td></tr>
<tr><td style="text-align:center;">CONDITIONS</td><td style="text-align:center;">PERFORMANCE</td></tr>
<tr><td>When given . . .</td><td>Students will . . .</td></tr>
<tr><td>

(Regarding Entire Responsibility:)

1. Written cases describing general appearance of arm circumference, and/or answers to questions about child's eating habits . . .

(Regarding Isolated Components:)

2.
</td><td>

. . . decide whether to refer each as a probable case of PCM.
</td></tr>
</table>

(Illustration 12-B, continued)

Course Title: Health Care Principles
For Day-Care Directors

ANALYZED RESPONSIBILITY

Responsibility: Identifies probable cases of protein calorie malnutrition (PCM) for referral to local health officer.

SKILLS	KNOWLEDGE	ATTITUDES

1. Observes children for one or more clinical signs. Looks at:
 	
— general energy level
— condition of arms, legs, belly, and face
— color of the hair.
	(1) Clinical signs of PCM:
	
	  a. marked weakness or inactivity
	  b. skinny arms and legs
	  c. pot belly (could also be worms)
	  d. puffy eyes, face, arms or legs
	  e. hair color changes from black to reddish brown.
		(1) Awareness of prevalence or PCM and consequences of failing to treat it.

2. Measures arm circumference to determine if lower than standard:
 	
  a. has child bend arm at elbow
  b. locates midpoint of upper arm
  c. has child relax arm at side
  d. determines if circumference at midpoint is 12cm or less.
	(2) How arm circumference test works:
	
	— Upper arm is made of a bone wrapped in muscle, fat and skin.
	— Narrowest place on bone is midpoint.
	— 12cm or less indicates serious fat loss and/or muscle wasting.
		(2) Handles and talks to child gently so as not to alarm him or her.

3. Takes diet history from mother or sibling who comes to pick up child. Asks: — if child is growing as well as others in the family — what foods child eats/likes — how "well" the child eats.	(3) Major sources of protein and calories in the foods eaten in village (diet information obtained in this way is rarely accurate, only a gross indicator).	(3) Questions mother or sibling in a casual nonthreatening way.

4. Decides whether to report a given child to local health officer as a probable case of PCM.	(4) Criteria for decision: Any one or combination of:
	
	  a. presence of clinical sign(s)
	  b. arm circumference of 12cm or less
	  c. suspicion that child not eating sufficient protein and calories.
	
	Background Theory —Sequence of events resulting in PCM: inadequate nutritional intake → loss of fat → muscle wasting → one or more clinical signs.	

(Illustration 12-B, continued)

PROFESSIONAL, TERMINAL, AND ENTRY COMPETENCIES

Responsibility: Identifies probable cases of protein calorie malnutrition (PCM) for referral to local health officers.

CONDITIONS	PERFORMANCE
Professional Competency: When given children in rural day-care centers which they are directing . . .	. . . practitioners observe children for clinical signs, measure arm circumference, take diet histories, and decide whether to report child as a probable case of PCM.
Terminal Student Competency: When given color slides of both well and malnourished children with written diet and arm-circumference data on each . . .	. . . students will select those with probable cases of PCM.
Entry Student Competencies: When given . . .	Students will . . .
(a) . . . a list of clinical signs of PCM and color slides of children manifesting one or more of these signs . . .	. . . recognize which clinical signs are exhibited by each child with PCM.
(b) . . . a tape measure and a cylinder . . .	. . . measure circumference of the cylinder.
(c) . . . a list of nutritional elements, nutritional functions, and common sources of each element . . .	. . . match each nutritional element to its respective function and source.
(d) . . . directions . . .	. . . list the most common staple foods eaten in their own villages.
(e) . . . hypothetical situation of having a seriously ill or injured child at day-care center they are directing . . .	. . . indicate referral to the local health officer as an option.

(Illustration 12-B, continued)

Course Title: Health Care Principles
for Day-Care Directors

INTERMEDIATE COMPETENCIES

Responsibility: Identifies probable cases of PCM for referral to local health officers.

CONDITIONS	PERFORMANCE
When given . . .	Students will . . .

(Regarding Entire Responsibility:)	
1. Written cases describing general appearance of arm circumference, and/or answers to questions about child's eating habits	. . . decide whether to refer each as a probable case of PCM.
(Regarding Isolated Components:)	
2. List of clinical signs, some associated with PCM and others not. . . .	. . . identify those signs which could indicate PCM.
3. Fellow student and measuring tape (in centimeters). . . .	. . . measure arm circumference, as if fellow student were a child.
4. Directions. . . .	. . . recall 12cm (or less) as critical point for a child's arm circumference.
5. Fellow student primed with a scenario. . . .	. . . take diet history.
6. Diet information for a variety of cases. . . .	. . . identify cases where child probably *not* getting enough protein and calories.
7. Multiple-choice items. . . .	. . . recognize:
	(a) prevalence of PCM
	(b) causes of PCM
	(c) stages of development
	(d) treatment for PCM
	(e) primary nutritional content of basic foods.

GUIDELINES FOR SOLVING PROBLEM 12

PROBLEM 12
How does one develop a set of intermediate competencies for a unit of instruction?

GUIDELINES

1. *Regarding the Entire Responsibility.* Design competencies only for those intermediate levels of simulation at which it will be both profitable and feasible for students to practice on their way to the terminal competency.

2. *Regarding Isolated Components.* Systematically review each skill, knowledge, and attitude component of each analyzed responsibility. As you consider each component, ask yourself:

   - Is this component adequately covered by one or more of the intermediate competencies regarding the entire responsibility? If not, do I want to include this component as an isolated competency?

   - Must students know or be able to do this before they can perform at one of the levels of simulation for the overall responsibility? If so, do I want to cover this component in isolation *before* including it with others?

   - If students fail at one of the higher levels of simulation, will I know if this component is responsible?

3. After deciding that a particular component should be covered by a competency, develop conditions and performance specifications for it by asking yourself:

   - How will I know that students know or can do this?

   - What should be provided for students by way of test conditions and what performance should be expected of students under those conditions?

   - Do these conditions and performance simulate the real-world conditions and performance as closely as possible, considering they are isolated from their logical context?

PROBLEM 13

How Does One Design Instructional Activities?

Once the intermediate competencies have been defined, the next problem is how to design instructional activities that will not only facilitate student learning of those competencies but also will be enjoyable for both students and instructor. Here experience with different methods and media is valuable, both in broadening one's range of possible ways to meet a given instructional function and in providing a basis for judging the probable success of a given activity with a given group of students. However, even without extensive experience, excellent instructional units can be developed by following a few guidelines.

The materials in this section review some of the guidelines provided in Chapter 3, where this aspect of the course design model was initially described, and also:

(a) demonstrate a step-by-step process for designing a set of activities for a single intermediate competency, and

(b) allow you a chance to analyze a complete instructional unit that was designed from a set of intermediate competencies.

DIRECTORY

TYPE OF PROBLEM	RELATED ILLUSTRATION	SEE PAGE
A step-by-step process	13-A. A Model Advocate Dialogue: Constructing a Family Tree	B-114
Analyzing an instructional unit	13-B. A Feedback Exercise: Industrial Hygiene	B-118
Summary	Guidelines for Solving Problem 13	B-129

ILLUSTRATION 13-A

A MODEL ADVOCATE DIALOGUE: CONSTRUCTING A FAMILY TREE

INSTRUCTIONAL SITUATION

One of the intermediate competencies for the course on pediatric paramedical care used as an example throughout Part A is as follows:

When given . . .	Students will . . .
Three generations of a family . . .	. . . construct a medical family tree.

Model Advocate: What instructional activities could you provide to facilitate your students' learning how to construct a three-generation family tree?

Instructor: That's easy; I'll give them a lecture. First I'll explain the importance of having a graphic summary of the entire family's medical situation, then I'll summarize the history of family tree use and conclude by telling them how to construct such a tree.

Model Advocate: And after your lecture is over, do you think your students will be able to actually construct such a tree?

Instructor: Humm . . . well maybe I should **show** them how to do it as well as talk about it. Sure, I'll demonstrate the process on the blackboard . . . say, isn't that one of those . . . what do you call them . . . **instructional functions**?

Model Advocate: Yes, and demonstrating the procedure is an excellent idea. But what about the other instructional functions. Perhaps you should consider each of them to see if any others are necessary here. What about *providing a frame of reference?* Won't these students need to know in what context they will be constructing family trees?

Instructor: That's why I was going to lecture on the history of family trees . . .to provide a historical context.

Model Advocate: Do you think this historical context will help the student understand why she is learning about family trees and when she will need to construct one? The only context your students need to have at this point is the medical interview.

Instructor: Oh, you mean I should show them how family trees are used in the taking of a medical history . . . I know, I could begin by showing them what a family tree looks like on a completed history form. That would also be a good time to explain how to interpret a tree; you know, circles stand for females, squares for males, and so on.

(Illustration 13-A, continued)

Model Advocate: That sounds like a better way to provide a frame of reference. Now what about the next function on the checklist: **providing a reason to learn**. Are you sure lecturing on the importance of using a family tree is the best way to initiate motivation here? As a general rule, it's a good idea to have students actively involved in the learning process whenever possible. Won't your students have enough background in these matters to discover on their own why such a medical family tree is a useful device?

Instructor: Sure, I can ask **them** why they think the family tree might be important and how it could be useful later on!

Model Advocate: Fine. The next function is often overlooked but very important when designing instructional activities . . . **shaping student attitudes**. Are there any particular attitudes related to this process of constructing trees that need to be conveyed?

Instructor: Well, often people are reluctant to talk about their family's medical problems. Some people feel it reflects badly on them and their family if say, their mother had epilepsy or whatever.

Model Advocate: So what should be done to convey the need for sensitivity on the part of the pediatric paramedic at this point in the interview?

Instructor: Maybe I could point out this potential problem when I first show students a family tree on a completed history form . . . the whole purpose of the tree is to spell out clearly who's got what and how they are related to each other genetically.

Model Advocate: What about including a "role reversal" as part of your demonstration of the actual construction process. Instead of providing case information, ask for a volunteer. Have that volunteering student play the role of a parent having to divulge her own family's medical history while you construct the tree on the blackboard. When you have finished, you can ask the student how she feels about having her family's medical problems laid out so clearly in black and white. Even if it doesn't bother **her**, the other students should be able to empathize and thereby understand the need to be sensitive and yet professional during this part of the history taking.

Instructor: That sounds like a good idea. I'll try it. What's next?

Model Advocate: **Transmitting information**. What knowledge components will these students need before they will be ready to construct a family tree and how will you provide these?

Instructor: Let's see now . . . once they can interpret the various symbols, all they really need to know is how to proceed. It's really very easy. I can explain everything as I demonstrate the process on the blackboard.

(Illustration 13-A, continued)

Model Advocate: Is the procedure simple enough that students will be ready to construct such a tree after a single demonstration, or will it be necessary to **allow students to practice** in order to assure successful performance during an actual interview situation.

Instructor: Well, the basic procedure is simple enough, but some cases do get complex. Often the information is not given in any logical order and has to be unscrambled. It's not always easy. Perhaps I could develop some cases where the data is scrambled and have students practice unraveling the information in the form of family trees.

Model Advocate: Will students be able to work on one of your case histories after a single demonstration, or will they also need some guidance such as a prompt sheet to remind them of the procedures?

Instructor: Oh, some guidance would be very helpful, particularly in the beginning. I can easily write up a series of guidelines on a single page. And perhaps I should show them how to use this guide sheet when I demonstrate the process the first time!

Model Advocate: Great idea! The best way to teach students to follow any guidelines you prepare is to model their use. Now what about practice at different levels of simulation. Will working on your canned cases be sufficient to prepare students to construct family trees in the midst of live interviews?

Instructor: Later on in the course I plan to have students practice filling in a blank history form during canned audiotaped interviews and then during actual interviews with classmates. By the time students work with live interviews situations, I'm pretty sure they will be able to handle the family tree construction.

Model Advocate: Good. Now what about the last function: **Providing feedback on student progress.** How will students know if the family trees they are constructing are right?

Instructor: Well, after having them unscramble the family data during their practice, I can ask for volunteers to write their versions on the blackboard. Then everyone can compare and even suggest alternate versions if there are any. Later on during higher level of simulations, I'll provide model answers whenever possible. I think the most crucial time for this feedback, however, is at the beginning, when they are developing the basic procedure.

Model Advocate: So now you are ready to summarize your set of instructional activities for this checkpoint.

(Illustration 13-A, continued)

Course Title: Pediatric
Paramedical Care

INSTRUCTIONAL UNIT

Responsibility No. 1: Takes a complete medical history from parents when appropriate.

COMPETENCIES	INSTRUCTIONAL ACTIVITIES
Given three generations of a family, students will construct a *medical family tree.*	— Show students a family tree on completed history form and explain symbols. Ask students about potential importance of this graphic form. — Using guide sheet, demonstrate the construction of a medical family tree (for a student volunteer). — Have students practice constructing family trees and comparing results on blackboards, using the same guide sheet.

ILLUSTRATION 13-B

A FEEDBACK EXERCISE: INDUSTRIAL HYGIENE

INTRODUCTION

See Illustration 9-B (page B-76) for background on this case.

In this exercise, you will be analyzing one of Dr. King's units of instruction and examining some of the decisions he made in designing these instructional activities.

During this exercise you will need to refer frequently to the following:

Analyzed Responsibility	Page B-122
Professional, Terminal and Entry Competencies	Page B-123
Intermediate Competencies	Page B-124
Instructional Unit	Page B-125

QUESTION 1

Review the analyzed responsibility (page B-122) and terminal and entry level competencies (page B-123); then study the intermediate competencies (page B-124), and finally read through the instructional activities (pages B-125 and B-126).

What items would you expect to find in Dr. King's prerequisite test to be administered before the course begins (see first instructional activity listed in the instructional unit page B-125)?

FEEDBACK

The entry student competencies listed on page B-123 represent a set of specifications for the test items in Dr. King's prerequisite test.

QUESTION 2

Has Dr. King included a posttest in his instructional unit? Where?

FEEDBACK

Yes . . . the last two activities, 16 and 17, represent the final level of simulation (i.e., terminal student competency) identified for this professional responsibility.

QUESTION 3

Did Dr. King include all of his intermediate competencies in this instructional unit? If not, which was/were omitted? **Suggestion:** Write the number of each intermediate competency (from page B-124) in the margin next to that activity which incorporates it.)

FEEDBACK

Intermediate Competency (IC) # 5 (interpreting environmental data) was omitted. The others should be matched as follows:

IC # 1 = Activity 15
IC # 2 = Activity 14
IC # 3 = Activity 11
IC # 4 = Activity 9
IC # 6 = Activity 12
IC # 7 = Activity 7

(Illustration 13-B, continued)

QUESTION 4	What could result from omitting IC # 5? Where in the list of instructional activities should it have been incorporated?

FEEDBACK   Students will learn to calibrate and operate the detection equipment, but they may not be able to interpret the resulting data in terms of health and safety hazards. Activities related to IC # 5 should probably be incorporated between instructional activities 9 and 10. However, some might prefer to teach data interpretation before the operation of the equipment used to obtain this data.

QUESTION 5   Why do you think Dr. King used his first intermediate level of simulation (videotaped tour) both at the beginning (activity 2) and end (activity 15) of this instructional unit? That is, what **instructional functions** are being served by each use of a videotaped tour?

INSTRUCTIONAL FUNCTIONS

1. Providing a frame of reference.
2. Providing a reason to learn.
3. Shaping student attitudes.
4. Transmitting information.
5. Demonstrating skills to be learned.
6. Allowing students to practice.
7. Providing feedback on student progress.

FEEDBACK   In activity 15, the videotaped tour helps prepare students for the terminal competency (i.e., a live industrial setting) by permitting them to practice and receive feedback at a high level of simulation within the classroom. However, in activity 2, the videotaped tour serves partly to provide a frame of reference for the entire unit (by showing students where the unit is headed), partly to provide a reason to learn (by challenging them with the critical issues to be focused on later) and, perhaps, partly as a type of pretest (by providing Dr. King with some idea of how much students already know about identifying hazards).

QUESTION 6   Instructional activities 4 to 7 are designed to prepare students for IC #7 (i.e., develop a legal intervention plan). What instructional functions are being met by each of these activities? (**Note**: A single activity can serve more than one instructional function.)

(Illustration 13-B, continued)

FEEDBACK

Activity 4: Transmitting information.

Activity 5: The primary function served by this activity is probably shaping student attitudes. However, also, this activity probably serves to some extent the instructional functions of providing a frame of reference and a reason to learn. Undoubtedly, certain information will also be transmitted and some student practice and feedback will occur; however, this information, practice, and feedback may not be related to the checkpoint performance (developing a legal intervention plan).

Activity 7: Allowing students to practice and providing feedback on student progress.

QUESTION 7

Has Dr. King included in his instructional unit all the **skill** and **knowledge** components listed in his analyzed responsibility? If not, which are missing? Do you think Dr. King has incorporated sufficient activities to convey each of the desired **attitudes** listed in this same analyzed responsibility?

FEEDBACK

A. Skills: All appear to be covered.

B. **Knowledge:** All appear to be covered except item 3 (interpretation of environmental data) which is related to the missing IC #5. Item 8 (implications of local political climate) is not included directly, but Dr. King probably expects these political implications to be brought out during the guest panel discussion.

C. **Attitudes:**

1. The first attitude (i.e., importance of well-being of workers over cost of controls) will probably be conveyed indirectly by the development of a legal intervention plan in activity 7. Perhaps Dr. King also intends to model this attitude continuously as a working assumption of the course.
2. The guest panel is probably intended to help instill respect for the concerns of the different parties involved in a work situation. This assumes that mere exposure to live representatives of each viewpoint will elicit the desired respect.
3. The importance of compromise and alternate solutions does **not** seem to be a major aspect of any particular instructional activity. Perhaps in fact this attitude component does **not** belong under this responsibility of **identifying** hazards, but rather under a later responsibility in the mastery description, such as "recommends solutions to eliminate health and safety hazards" (see page B-76 for complete list of professional responsibilities for this course).

(Illustration 13-B, continued)

QUESTION 8   In general instructional activities are developed to facilitate student learning of the intermediate competencies. Dr. King has included all (but #5) of his intermediate competencies in this set of instructional activities. See if you can group the activities with their associated intermediate competencies. **Suggestion**: Draw lines between sets of activities related to the same intermediate competency.

FEEDBACK   See pages B-127 and B-128 for appropriate grouping of activities around each intermediate competency.

QUESTION 9   What do you think of Dr. King's sequence of intermediate competencies? Does it seem logical, or do you think there is a "better" order?

FEEDBACK   Dr. King did not simply teach all his component competencies first and then allow students to practice at the lower levels of simulation for the entire responsibility. Rather, he used his third intermediate competency (the matching of exercises) as a mechanism for students to review the relationships described in their reading assignments. Dr. King's sequence does appear to be a logical ordering of the intermediate competencies, but others are certainly possible; for example,

Intermediate Competency:

4	(calibrating and operating monitoring equipment)
5	(interpretation of data from monitoring equipment)
6	(interpretation of medical and safety records)
7	(developing a legal intervention plan)
3	(matching exercise)
2	(incomplete case study)
1	(videotaped tour)

(Illustration 13-B, continued)

ANALYZED RESPONSIBILITY

Responsibility No. 3: Identifies health and safety hazards in industrial settings.

A. *Skills:*

1. Observes the workers, processes, equipment, products, and by-products.
2. Records observations as related to health and safety hazards.
3. Measures and records physical parameters: sound levels, dust, solvents, etc.
4. Analyzes medical and safety records of workers.
5. Recognizes health and safety hazards from above data.

B. *Knowledge:*

1. Methods of observation and recording, including checklists, interview technique, audio- and videotape, diaries, and standard government forms.
2. Operation and calibration of environmental detection equipment.
3. Interpretation of environmental data.
4. Interpretation of medical and accident records.
5. Laws and regulations (a) governing the health and safety of industrial workers, and (b) defining the responsibilities and authority of inspectors.
6. Safety hazards by work type.
7. Health hazards, noise, dust, solvents, irritants, etc.
8. Implications of local political climate (the concerns and interactions of management, unions, and workers).

C. *Attitudes:*

1. Physical and psychological well-being of industrial workers is more important than cost of controls.
2. Respect for the concerns of management, union leaders, and workers.
3. Importance of compromise and alternate solutions if immediate changes are not feasible.

(Illustration 13-B, continued)

Course Title: Industrial Hygiene

PROFESSIONAL, TERMINAL AND ENTRY COMPETENCIES

Responsibility No. 3: Identifies health and safety hazards in industrial settings.

CONDITIONS	PERFORMANCE
Professional Competency: When given access to a variety of industrial settings for individual observation, acccess to environmental detection equipment for wide range of harmful agents, and to medical records of workers . . .	. . . practitioners observe workers, record observations, measure physical parameters, analyze medical records, and identify with documentation the health and safety hazards of each setting.
Terminal Student Competency: When given a guided group tour of an industrial setting with access to limited detection equipment and to medical records of the workers . . .	. . . students will observe workers, record observations, measure physical parameters, indicate what additional equipment is desirable, analyze medical records, and identify with documentation the health and safety hazards of that setting . . . write individual report explaining what other workers and processes should have been observed and any other limitations of the study.
Entry Student Competencies: When given . . . (a) a list of harmful industrial agents . . . (b) a list of terms (such as calibrate, toxic, etc.) . . . (c) a set of lung X-rays, some diseased, some not . . . (d) checklists for observing three sets of simple procedures . . .	Students will . . . . . . identify body system affected (80% accuracy). . . . define correctly 75% of the terms. . . . identify diseased lungs (at rate of 1 X-ray/min.). . . . use the checklist while observing videotapes of the procedures being performed (in three different settings).

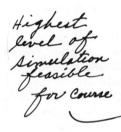

Highest level of simulation feasible for Course

(Illustration 13-B, continued)

Course Title: Industrial
Hygiene

INTERMEDIATE COMPETENCIES

Responsibility: Identifies health and safety hazards in industrial settings.

CONDITIONS	PERFORMANCE
When given . . .	Students will . . .

(Regarding Entire Responsibility:)

1. Videotaped tour of an industrial setting, and an incomplete set of data regarding potentially harmful agents and medical and accident records . . .

   . . . record observations of taped workers, specify what other observations and data are needed but missing, and identify potential health and safety hazards.

2. A case study of an industrial setting including an incomplete set of data . . .

   . . . specify a plan for observation, which data are relevant, which are missing, and what potential hazards should be documented.

3. Separate lists of (a) types of industries, (b) potential hazards, (c) types of work-related diseases and injuries, (d) physical parameters, and (e) environmental detection equipment . . .

   . . . match industries with potential hazards; hazards with related diseases and injuries; diseases and injuries with related physical parameters; and physical parameters with associated detection equipment.

(Regarding Isolated Components:)

4. Environmental monitoring equipment in lab setting . . .

   . . . calibrate accurately and operate within limitation of equipment.

5. Environmental data collected from various detection equipment in a variety of settings . . .

   . . . identify health and safety hazards.

6. Medical and safety records of industrial settings . . .

   . . . identify possible causes of disease or injury.

7. Open-ended film depicting plight of workers where management is apparently winning . . .

   . . . develop a legal intervention plan whereby an industrial hygienist helps the workers.

(Illustration 13-B, continued)

	Course Title: Industrial Hygiene
INSTRUCTIONAL UNIT	

Responsibility No. 3: Identifies health and safety hazards in industrial settings.

COMPETENCIES	INSTRUCTIONAL ACTIVITIES
	1. Administer prerequisite test prior to course admission. Suggest remedial action for those who failed any parts of prerequisite test.
	2. Show videotaped tour of an industry; and hand out set of data regarding the health, safety, and environment of the workers in that industry. After videotape, have class discussion during which you ask randomly selected students to try to identify potential hazards, determine what additional information is needed, and suggest possible ways to obtain this information.
	3. Have students read handout describing typical methods of observing workers and recording information possibly related to health and safety hazards.
	4. Have students read synopses of laws and regulations governing industrial workers.
	5. Have students debate and discuss with panel of guests the interpretation and application of new federal laws to different types of hypothetical industrial settings. Guests to include state industrial hygienist, manager of a local industry, local union leader, and representative of an insurance company.
	6. Show an open-ended film depicting the plight of foundry workers (exposed to stresses of heat, sound, dust, etc). In film, management appears to be winning with complaints of high cost of controls and maintenance.
	7. In groups of three, have students develop legal intervention plans whereby an industrial hygienist helps the workers in the foundry. Have group leaders present final plans of each small group for whole-class discussion and feedback. (Have lawyer present for this final discussion.)
	8. Demonstrate the use of environmental monitoring equipment. Discuss limitations and sources of error.
	9. Have students practice using and calibrating the different types of equipment in lab setting. [Lab exercises emphasize (a) need for careful calibration, and (b) limitations of equipment.]
	10. Students read two chapters in textbook describing specific health and safety hazards by type of industry and ways to detect and measure effects of these hazards.
	11. Turn in open-book progress test in which students match industries with potential hazards, hazards with related diseases and injuries, diseases and injuries with related physical parameters, and physical parameters with associated detection equipment.

Table continued on next page

(Illustration 13-B, continued)

12. In pairs (preferably physician with nonphysician), students identify possible causes of disease or injury in series of short case problems involving the medical and safety records of different industrial settings. Afterwards, whole class compares answers.

13. Have class work together on identifying the health and safety hazards for a complete case study. Demonstrate method of documenting these hazards with available data.

14. Have students develop plans for observation when given a case study of an industrial setting along with incomplete data. Have them also specify what data is missing and what potential hazards should be documented.

15. Show videotaped tour of a second industry, and hand out a set of data regarding potentially harmful agents and medical and accident records. Have students practice observing the workers and recording their observations. As a class, have them specify what other observations and data are needed but missing from the videotape, and also to identify potential health and safety hazards.

16. Working in teams of four, arrange for students to have a guided group tour of a local industrial setting with access to limited detection equipment and the medical and safety records of workers. Each team is responsible for observing workers, recording their observations, measuring available physical parameters, and analyzing medical records.

17. Each individual student responsible for turning in a final report of the study, identifying potential health and safety hazards with documentation, and specifying what other observations and data should have been made if possible.

(Illustration 13-B, continued)

Course Title: Industrial Hygiene

INSTRUCTIONAL UNIT

Responsibility No. 3: Identifies health and safety hazards in industrial settings.

COMPETENCIES	INSTRUCTIONAL ACTIVITIES
Prerequisite test *Introduction to unit* *Not related to any specific checkpoint*	1. Administer prerequisite test prior to course admission. Suggest remedial action for those who failed any parts of prerequisite test. 2. Show videotaped tour of an industry, and hand out set of data regarding the health, safety, and environment of the workers in that industry. After videotape, have class discussion during which you ask randomly selected students to try to identify potential hazards, determine what additional information is needed, and suggest possible ways to obtain this information. 3. Have students read handout describing typical methods of observing workers and recording information possibly related to health and safety hazards.
IC #7	4. Have students read synopses of laws and regulations governing industrial workers. 5. Have students debate and discuss with panel of guests the interpretation and application of new federal laws to different types of hypothetical industrial settings. Guests to include state industrial hygienist, manager of a local industry, local union leader, and representative of an insurance company. 6. Show an open-ended film depicting the plight of foundry workers (exposed to stresses of heat, sound, dust, etc). In film, management appears to be winning with complaints of high cost of controls and maintenance. 7. In groups of three, have students develop legal intervention plans whereby an industrial hygienist helps the workers in the foundry. Have group leaders present final plans of each small group for whole-class discussion and feedback. (Have lawyer present for this final discussion.)
IC #4	8. Demonstrate the use of environmental monitoring equipment. Discuss limitations and sources of error. 9. Have students practice using and calibrating the different types of equipment in lab setting. [Lab exercises emphasize (a) need for careful calibration, and (b) limitations of equipment.]

Table continued on next page

(Illustration 13-B, continued)

IC #3	10. Students read two chapters in textbook describing specific health and safety hazards by type of industry and ways to detect and measure effects of these hazards. 11. Turn in open-book progress test in which students match industries with potential hazards, hazards with related diseases and injuries, diseases and injuries with related physical parameters, and physical parameters with associated detection equipment.
IC #6	12. In pairs (preferably physician with nonphysician), students identify possible causes of disease or injury in series of short case problems involving the medical and safety records of different industrial settings. Afterward, whole class compares answers.
IC #2	13. Have class work together on identifying the health and safety hazards for a complete case study. Demonstrate method of documenting these hazards with available data. 14. Have students develop plans for observation when given a a case study of an industrial setting along with incomplete data. Have them also specify what data is missing and what potential hazards should be documented.
IC #1	15. Show videotaped tour of a second industry, and hand out a set of data regarding potentially harmful agents and medical and accident records. Have students practice observing the workers and recording their observations. As a class, have them specify what other observations and data are needed but missing from the videotape, and also to identify potential health and safety hazards.
Terminal Competency *(Posttest)*	16. Working in teams of four, arrange for students to have a guided group tour of a local industrial setting with access to limited detection equipment and the medical and safety records of workers. Each team is responsible for observing workers, recording their observations, measuring available physical parameters, and analyzing medical records. 17. Each individual student is responsible for turning in a final report of the study, identifying potential health and safety hazards with documentation, and specifying what other observations and data should have been made if possible.

GUIDELINES FOR SOLVING PROBLEM 13

PROBLEM 13   Is there a "best" way to develop instructional activities for a unit of instruction?

GUIDELINES

1. *Use the list of instructional functions as a checklist:*

   (a) Review **each** instructional function before finalizing a set of instructional activities for a given intermediate competency.
   (b) Often several instructional functions can be met simultaneously by the same instructional activity.

2. *Check instructional units for completeness:*

   (a) Be sure all *Intermediate competencies* have been included in a unit of instruction for a given responsibility (unless you later discover that certain competencies were not necessary after all).
   (b) Be sure all skill, knowledge, and attitude **components** have been included in a unit of instruction for a given responsibility. Watch especially for components not covered by intermediate competencies, such as attitudes (since attitudes are rarely incorporated as competencies).

3. *Be aware of the effects of sequencing:*

   (a) Usually there is no single best way for a series of instructional activities to be sequenced.
   (b) Select a logical order that allows prerequisites to be met at the appropriate times but provides variety and challenge early in the unit.
   (c) Beginning a unit with an illustration at a reasonably high level of simulation is a particularly good way to provide both a frame of reference and a reason to learn.

PROBLEM 14

Why Choose One Instructional Method or Medium Over Another?

INTRODUCTION Teachers must select instructional methods and media whenever they are planning instructional activities for specific intermediate and terminal student competencies. At these times teachers often ask for guidance in determining the "best" method/media for their particular situations.

Unfortunately, there are no decisive rules for this selection process. Experimental research in the area indicates that, when students know what is expected of them, they tend to learn regardless of the teaching methods/media used. Nonetheless, **some** method and/or media generally must be selected, and consideration of certain instructional, motivational, and administrative issues may be helpful.

The materials in this section are designed to demonstrate and provide practice with these issues to be considered when selecting methods and media.

NOTE: Before continuing with this section, read or review Chapter 9 (beginning on page C-54) which describes the various methods and media dealt within this section.

DIRECTORY

TYPE OF PROBLEM	RELATED ILLUSTRATION	SEE PAGE
What is the difference between a method and a medium?	14-A. Definitions	B-131
How to determine appropriate instructional methods/media?	14-B. A Feedback Exercise: Selecting Methods and Media	B-132
Summary	Guidelines for Solving Problem 14	B-136

ILLUSTRATION 14-A

DEFINITIONS

INTRODUCTION   Certain terms are used repeatedly when discussing instructional methods and media. It is important to understand the distinctions between them.

DEFINITIONS   *Method*—a type of instructional activity, such as role playing, group discussion, or a guest interview.

Medium—the vehicle or channel through/by which information is transmitted, such as film, videotape, slides, or the spoken word.

NOTE: In most instances, a particular method involves the use of specific media. For example, role playing is a method in which information is conveyed through several media—spoken word, bodily and facial movement, and sometimes even touch. However, the distinction between method and medium becomes trivial in some instances: that is, showing a film is a method where film is the medium; or lecturing is a method where the spoken word is the medium.

Hardware—Equipment, such as film projectors, tape recorders, or computers.

Software—Whatever the equipment transmits, such as the film, the audiotape, or the computer program.

NOTE: Most methods and media involve both hardware and software. For example, the showing-a-film method utilizes a film projector and screen (hardware) and a film (software); the lecture method utilizes a lecturer (hardware) and his/her fund of information and skills (software).

ILLUSTRATION 14-B

A FEEDBACK EXERCISE: SELECTING METHODS AND MEDIA

INTRODUCTION   In general, when selecting methods and media, one should consider:

(a) *instructional factors* such as:

– the extent to which the conditions and student performance provided by the method/media match those of the competency to be learned, and

the extent to which the method/media provides for the instructional functions to be served; for example, practice and feedback.

(b) *motivational factors* such as:

– the need for variety or special effects to arouse or maintain student interest, and

– differences in student learning styles.

(c) *administrative factors* such as:

– availability of both hardware and software
– feasibility of implementing the method or media.

QUESTION 1   Your instructional objective is for 75 medical students to be able to interpret the reported results of a CBC (Complete Blood Count). Which of the following methods/media is most appropriate and why?

a. Explanation in textbook followed by a lecture with chalkboard as the only visual medium.
b. Interactive lecture-demonstration with slides of actual CBC reports, followed by practice in small groups with copies of CBC reports.
c. Videotape presentation describing a series of actual cases and including the interpretation of CBC reports for each case.
d. A color film on how to interpret a CBC report, followed by a class discussion of the film.

FEEDBACK   a. *Textbook and Lecture:* Not the best choice, since the conditions and performance provided by the media do not match those of the terminal competency. Conditions for interpreting CBC reports would involve the presence of such reports. Although a textbook or handout may provide examples of these reports, they are not likely to require students to practice interpreting them. Similarly the lecture method does not lend itself to student practice and feedback unless the lecture is programmed. And even if the lecture

(Illustration 14-B, continued)

were programmed to allow students to practice interpreting CBC reports, the chalkboard is probably not the best medium for displaying a series of these reports. Slides, flipchart, or overhead projections would be better.

b. *Slides and Copies:* Probably the best choice since both the conditions and student performance is in the same medium as required by the terminal competency. There is adequate opportunity for students to practice and receive feedback; and the projected slides will probably produce sufficiently large images for the students to read the reports to be interpreted.

c and d. *Videotape and Film:* Usually there is little point in using media more complex than required by the behavior to be learned. Since visual motion (and color) are not crucial parts of interpreting a printed report, neither a videotape nor a color film is the most cost-effective medium to use. Not only are they generally more expensive to produce or purchase, but student participation and feedback may be hampered. In addition, videotapes are difficult to view in large classrooms unless several TV monitors are strategicly placed around the room. **Note:** If a film or videotape happens to be available and is at least accurate, the instructor could suggest that students view it at their own option, either in addition to or in lieu of attending class demonstrations.

QUESTION 2

Methods/media such as group discussion, programmed texts, and the case method provide ample opportunity for students to interact with the instruction and receive feedback. Films, reference texts, and lectures, on the other hand, are more likely to place students in a passive role. In general, the more opportunity for students to respond and receive feedback, the more effective the learning.

How can noninteractive methods and media (such as films, lectures, reference textbooks, etc.) be supplemented to provide opportunities for more active participation on the part of students?

FEEDBACK

Listed below are a few of the more common techniques used to increase the interactive quality of methods and media:

1. Providing students with a list of questions to accompany a film, lecture, or text assignment.
2. Stopping a film or videotape at certain points and having students react or answer questions.
3. Encouraging students to interrupt a lecture whenever they have questions, rather than hold questions until the end.

(Illustration 14-B, continued)

4. Developing an adjunct program to accompany a reference text (see Adjunct Programs, page C-105).

5. Changing from the lecture format to the programmed lecture format (see Programmed Lectures, page C-76).

QUESTION 3

Some students may have special difficulty learning effectively from certain types of media. In general, which media in the right-hand column below do you think would be better suited to the students described in the left-hand column?

____1. Students whose native language is different from that used in the instructional process.

    a. Videotape or film

____2. Students who grew up watching television every day.

    b. Lectures with slides

____3. Poor readers

    c. Textbooks or handouts

FEEDBACK

1-c Foreign-speaking students often have more difficulty with audio presentations than with written materials. Lectures and films sometimes have to be supplemented extensively with readings or handouts.

2-a The "TV generation" tend to be more visually oriented than persons not raised with TV. Thus they generally learn better from pictures than from words, particularly written words. (Lecture with slides would also be acceptable media for these students.)

3-b (or a) Poor readers generally learn more efficiently from audiovisual presentations than from printed materials.

QUESTION 4

After each method or medium listed below, circle "yes," "no," or "perhaps," to indicate whether it should be included in a unit of instruction designed to teach 50 medical students to interpret moving ECG (electrocardiograph) records on an oscilloscope.

a. Simplified line drawings of ECG records shown with overhead projector   yes   no   perhaps

b. 35mm slides of clear, noise-free typical records shown on a large screen   yes   no   perhaps

c. Xerox copies of actual records of varying clarity   yes   no   perhaps

d. Class demonstration with actual oscilloscope   yes   no   perhaps

(Illustration 14-B, continued)

e. Film or videotape on how to interpret
moving ECG records   yes   no   perhaps

f. Lab exercise in which students practice
with actual oscilloscopes   yes   no   perhaps

FEEDBACK

a, b, and c: Perhaps. Each of these involves a **static** ECG record whereas the terminal competency involves a **moving** record. However, depending on the entry level of the students, one or more of these visual media may be appropriate. If students have had no previous experience with ECG records, exposing them to moving records may hopelessly confuse them. Even static ECG records may be too difficult to handle if they are not clear or contain too many rare phenomena. Thus one might use all three media in succession, beginning with line drawings to teach the basic discriminations and gradually progressing to more difficult discriminations.

d: No. Not appropriate for large class, since students sitting at the back of the room would not be able to see.

e: Yes: Probably a good way to demonstrate the process of interpreting moving graphs to a large class. Film would be better than videotape unless several TV monitors are available.

f: Yes. Live practice is essential for learning this competency.

GUIDELINES FOR SOLVING PROBLEM 14

PROBLEM 14 | Why choose one method or medium over another when designing instruction for a particular competency?

GUIDELINES | Ask yourself the following questions when selecting from alternative instructional methods and media:

Instructional Issues

- Do the conditions and student performance provided by the method/media match those of the competency to be learned?

- Does the method/media provide for the instructional functions that need to be met, for example, practice, feedback, demonstration, etc.?

Motivational Issues

- Is there a need for variety in methods/media to arouse or maintain student interest?

- Are there special student characteristics which indicate that some methods or media are more appropriate than others (e.g., language or reading problems)?

- Is it feasible to accommodate different learning styles by offering a choice of alternative methods or media for meeting the same instructional objective?

Administrative Issues

- Are materials (hardware and software) already available—or can they be borrowed, developed, or purchased at a reasonable cost?

- Can the method/media be used (operated, managed) and maintained (updated) easily?

- Does the learning environment permit adequate use of the method/media (e.g., noise level, space, lighting, electrical wiring, or patient considerations such as the right to privacy)?

- Is the quality of the medium adequate to illustrate critical features for the expected size of audience?

- Does the anticipated amount of use justify the initial costs?

  - Can the materials be used by others and the cost shared with them?

  - Are there less expensive methods/media that will do the job as well, or nearly as well?

  - Is a multi-media presentation being considered when a single medium would be perfectly adequate?

PROBLEM 15

How Does One Construct a Syllabus?

INTRODUCTION The last task in designing a course is putting all the instructional activities together into a course syllabus.

This section is designed to give you practice in constructing a syllabus for a set of instructional activities.

DIRECTORY

ILLUSTRATION 15-A

A MINI-CASE: INDUSTRIAL HYGIENE

INSTRUCTIONAL SITUATION

See Illustrations 9-B (page B-76) and 13-B (page B-118) for background on this case.

Dr. King is now ready to convert his instructional unit into part of his course syllabus.

Constraints:

(a) A two-hour block of time has been allotted to this course on Monday and Thursday mornings.
(b) Dr. King has determined that this portion of the course can take no more than four weeks if he is to cover all the other instructional units.
(c) Students may be expected to spend about an hour outside of class in preparation for every hour spent inside class.

QUESTION

Construct a partial syllabus from the instructional activities listed in Illustration 13-B on page B-118 (begin with activity 2, since the first activity describes the prerequisite test to be given before the class meets). Use the format suggested and modeled in Chapter 3 of Unit A.

Suggestion: Read the guidelines for solving Problem 15 (page B-137) before beginning.

FEEDBACK

Compare your syllabus to the one developed by Dr. King below. Some combinations and descriptions of activities may be different, but your syllabus should be similar to Dr. King's.

(Illustration 15-A, continued)

PARTIAL SYLLABUS

Course Title: Industrial Hygiene
Unit Title: Health and Safety Hazards

School of Public Health
1974-1975

Session	In-Class Activities	Assignment for Next Session
1 (2 hr) Monday	*Videotaped Tour:* Of an industry. Hand out relevant set of data. *Instructor-led Discussion:* Of potential hazards observed in videotape, additional information needed, etc. *Instructor-led Discussion:* Hand out materials describing methods of observing workers—go over handout as time permits.	Read handout on methods of observing workers and recording observations. Read handout summarizing laws and regulations governing industrial workers.
2 (2 hr) Thursday	*Guest Panel:* Have students and panel discuss and debate interpretation and application of new laws to series of hypothetical industrial settings.	Read Chapter 1 of textbook. (covering health and safety hazards by type of industry).
3 (2 hr) Monday	*Open-ended Film:* Depicting plight of foundry workers. *Small Groups:* Students develop legal intervention plans to help workers in groups of three. *Class Feedback:* Have small group leaders present final plans of each small group for whole class discussion and feedback (lawyer present if possible)	Read Chapter 2 in textbook. (covering ways to detect and measure effects of hazards).
4 (2 hr) Thursday	*Lab Demonstration:* Environmental monitoring equipment. Discuss limitations and sources of error. *Lab Exercises:* Practice in using and calibrating different types of equipment. *Instructor-led Discussion:* Interpretation of sets of data from different types of equipment.	Take-home open-book quiz. (series of matching items)

(Syllabus continued)

(Illustration 15-A, continued)

Session	In-Class Activities	Assignment for Next Session
5 (2 hr) Monday	*Review Quiz:* Go over quiz with whole class. *Exercise:* In pairs, students work on short cases involving medical and safety records of different factories. Practice identifying possible causes of diseases or injuries. *Class Feedback:* Have whole class compare solutions to cases.	Read complete case for Thursday's class discussion.
6 (2 hr) Thursday	*Instructor-led Discussion:* Identify health and safety hazards for a complete case study. *Demonstration:* Instructor demonstrates documentation of hazards.	Develop plans for observation when given a case study of an industrial setting along with incomplete data.
7 (2 hr) Monday	*Review:* Go over plans for observation developed as assignment. *Videotaped Tour:* Students practice observing, recording observations. *Instructor-led Discussion:* Specify other observations and data needed but missing from videotape. Also identify potential hazards.	Attend guided group tour of local industrial setting in groups of four. Observe workers, record observations, inspect medical and safety records, and measuring available physical parameters.
8 (2 hr) Thursday	No formal class meeting: Teams of students visiting same local industry should meet to exchange and compare data.	Prepare final report on health and safety hazards identified in guided group tour.
9 (2 hr) Monday	Turn in final report. (begin next unit)	

GUIDELINES FOR SOLVING PROBLEM 15

PROBLEM 15   How does one construct a syllabus from a set of instructional activities?

GUIDELINES

1. Set up a three-column syllabus worksheet with the following headings:

    — Session (or date if known)
    — In-class activities
    — Assignments for next session

2. Identify those activities that must take place **in class** and those that may be assigned **out of class**.

3. Give each activity an appropriate label for later reference purposes; mini-lecture, demonstration, exercise, small-group practice, instructor-led discussion, etc.

4. Try to visualize each session as you describe what it will include. Be sure the activities within each session are realistic in terms of the time limits.

PROBLEM 16

What About That First Class Session?

INTRODUCTION In general, this book does not extend the course design process to the level of writing specific session plans, designing handouts, writing test items, etc. However, the first session in any course is of such overriding importance to what happens in the rest of the course, that some guidelines are offered here regarding this initial contact with the students.

DIRECTORY

TYPE OF PROBLEM	RELATED ILLUSTRATION	SEE PAGE
How to begin the first session	16-A. A Mini-Case: Designing the First Session	B-143
Summary	Guidelines For Solving Problem 16	B-144

ILLUSTRATION 16-A

A MINI-CASE: DESIGNING THE FIRST SESSION

INSTRUCTIONAL SITUATION

Tomorrow is the first class session of the course Ms. Anderson has been preparing for three months. She described professional performance, terminal competencies and intermediate competencies before carefully planning the instructional activities for her nine-week course. But suddenly she realized that she is not sure how to get started in this first class session.

QUESTION

What types of things does Ms. Anderson need to consider and decide regarding this first session? That is, what kind of things will she need to do and say before the class gets started and during the first few minutes before any formal instructional activities are begun?

FEEDBACK

There are many things you could have listed, and those below are not inclusive. But some of the decisions that should be made involve:

(a) Seating arrangements
(b) The opening routine:
   – introductions?
   – roles to be played by students and instructor(s)?
   – overall structure of the course?
   – requirements for passing?
   – goals or objectives, etc.?
(c) Materials to be handed out and when?

The first session sets the norms and expectations for the entire course. It is important to realize that these norms and expectations are communicated in part by the **nonverbal messages** or implications of whatever you do or say overtly. The guidelines on the following pages attempt to point out the nature of the nonverbal messages communicated by alternative approaches to this first session.

GUIDELINES FOR SOLVING PROBLEM 16

PROBLEM 16	How does one design the first class session? What decisions need to be made and what are the implications of these decisions for the course?

GUIDELINES

1. *Decide on classroom seating arrangements.*

When students walk into a classroom for the first time, the way the seats are arranged tells them something about the session to come. For example:

Type of Seating	*Non Verbal Message*
(a) Chairs in rows facing instructor.	Instructor will speak; students will listen and probably **not** talk to each other very much.
(b) Chairs arranged in a circle; no special chair singled out for instructor.	It is important for everyone to see everyone else. Students will speak to each other.
(c) Chairs in large semicircle around instructor.	Instructor will lead but student-to-student communications may be important.
(d) Individual carrels separated by dividers.	Students will work alone with various instructional materials; nobody talks to anybody else.
(e) Sofas, chairs, coffee table, and rug.	Instruction will be relaxed and informal. Likely to be student-to-student communication.

2. *Determine opening routine.*

What you say and what activities you suggest at the very beginning of the session will influence the expectations of students. After **giving your name** and the **name of the course**, you may want to use an adaptation of one of these opening routines:

Opening Routine	*Non Verbal Message*
(a) *"The first thing for us to do is to get acquainted with each other. Then I'll outline my ideas for the course and get some feedback from you on your goals and interests. Let's begin by going around the room and introducing ourselves. Please also say something about your reasons for taking the course."*	– Instructor has goals and structure in mind but it's important for students to get to know one another first. – Student input is valued and course is flexible depending on student feedback.

(b) *"The first thing I'll do is outline the purposes, methods, and grading system; then I'll answer any questions you have before we get on with the first lesson."*

— Instructor will make the most important instructional decisions in this class.

— It's not important for students to interact with each other.

(c) *"I'd like to get some information from each of you on your backgrounds, interest in the course, and what you expect to be doing after the course. I'll tabulate this data here on the blackboard as you answer so we'll all know what resources we have to learn from."*

— Assumes that students are different and have valuable backgrounds to contribute to course.

— Sets expectation that we can all learn from each other.

— Sets expectation that student resources will be used later in the course.

— Assumes students will be interested in these variables.

3. *Outline your view of the roles to be played by instructor (s), students, other staff, etc.*

Students are very interested in what kind of person you are and what the course is going to be like. There are many different kinds of role expectations you can set up, depending on your preferences. You may wish to use an adaptation of one of these:

(a) *"When you leave here, you will have to be problem-solvers. You will be on your own in solving unstructured, open-ended problems. So this course will resemble your future situation. You'll be on your own a lot, discussing problems with fellow students and me, and coming up with solutions. I'll be available to help in any way I can . . ."*

— There will be very little structure to the course.

— Students can expect help and support from both instructor and fellow students.

— Students will do a lot of working on their own during the course.

(b) *"We are going to cover a great deal of material in this course. You will be taken through a series of planned experiences designed to get you to the point where you can perform like a professional. I've handed out a list of the objectives for the course. The exams will only be on these objectives. If you know these things, you'll do well. I don't mind giving all A's."*

— Student's role is to learn the material planned by the instructor.

— Instructor is precise and goals are known.

— Can expect to be tested only on what's covered.

— Instructor will help in case of difficulty with the course materials.

4. *Decide how to describe the course.*

There are many things you could say about the course depending on how it will be conducted and what expectations you wish students to have. You may want to use one or more of the following components:

(a) *"The requirements for passing this course and the grading system involve . . ."*

The instructor is forthright about what the standards are and how students will be evaluated.

(b) *"In general, assignments for homework will entail . . ."*

Instructor realizes importance of student time and gives realistic appraisal of what to expect.

(c) *"The first things we will do are . . ."*

Students are often unsure about beginning a new subject and feel more comfortable knowing what the structure will be.

(d) *"I've set aside some time in this first session for us to discuss your expectations of this course, what problems you anticipate, and what involvement you've had with this area in the past."*

— Sets up norm of responsiveness to student needs—a willingness to modify aspects of course to meet expressed student needs.

— Allows students to begin to "connect" with course purposes.

(e) *"My bias in this subject matter is . . ."*

— There are more than one points of view and instructor is not neutral.

(f) *"I hope you will find me open to discussion. I expect I will change some of my own ideas during this course."*

— The instructor's ideas can be challenged.

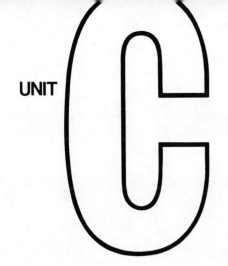

Methods to Facilitate Application

Unit C

METHODS TO FACILITATE APPLICATION

INTRODUCTION   Unit C specifies methods and techniques to implement the course design model. Each of the three chapters in Unit C is devoted to the application of one of the three phases of the model.

Unit C is intended as an introduction to these methods and techniques. Each is described only briefly, and annotated bibliographies are provided for those who wish a more detailed presentation.

Chapter 7

METHODS FOR PHASE 1: DESCRIBING PROFESSIONAL PERFORMANCE

This chapter contains brief descriptions of the nine methods of performance analysis listed below.

Contents

One or more of these techniques, or variations of them, can be used to analyze the requirements of almost any currently existing professional (or nonprofessional) role. Thus, they can be used to verify a mastery description, or in the absence of an original mastery description, to help an instructor develop one.

Additional details on these methods of performance analysis can be found in one or more of the annotated references included at the end of each section.

QUESTIONNAIRE

DESCRIPTION

The **questionnaire** technique involves having a large number of individuals fill out a specially devised form containing a series of questions. The questions on the questionnaire may be either open-ended or closed-ended:

> **Open-ended** questions ask respondents to write their answers in their own words; whereas

> **Closed-ended** questions ask respondents to select their answers from specified alternatives.

Usually a job questionnaire asks for information about the conditions under which the respondent works, and then, if open-ended, provides ample space for describing the position. Some questionnaires are more structured and contain a series of narrowly defined topics or types of responsibilities around which the respondent is asked to organize his description.

ADVANTAGES

- Can be used in a mail survey to obtain occupational information from widely scattered respondents.

- Can yield a large amount of data compared to the number of man-hours required of the originator.

- One of the least expensive methods in terms of both money and man-hours.

- Particularly good for higher level positions where people read and write easily.

- If well-structured, can be used to compare information from various respondents.

- Particularly good for collecting information about the use of concrete things, such as materials, tools, or equipment.

LIMITATIONS

- Percentage of returns is often inadequate and may represent a biased sample.

- Unless close-ended or highly structured, a heavy demand is placed on recall, resulting in many incomplete forms and forms lacking in the necessary detail.

- When activities are missing from a description, one does not know if the respondent does not do it or simply forgot to include it.

- Although data collection is relatively easy, organization and analysis of the essentially unstructured, handwritten information obtained from open-ended questionnaires is at best a difficult undertaking. (Data from closed-ended questionnaires can usually be analyzed by computers.)

- Responses to open-ended questions are sometimes ambiguous, and subjective decisions may be required to interpret and categorize the activities described. Closed-ended questions, on the other hand, may not include all the alternatives or may exclude the possibility of getting "new" types of responses.

EXAMPLE (AN OPEN-ENDED QUESTIONNAIRE)

NAME OF POSITION: PHYSICAL THERAPIST

1. Describe your working conditions (type of institution; physical setting, etc).

   _____

   _____

2. List your major responsibilities and describe briefly how you carry them out and what proportion of your total time they require.

Responsibilities	Explanation	Percent of Total Time

3. If you supervise the work of others, please describe the nature of the work supervised.

   _____

   _____

   _____

4. List any equipment or machines you use regularly, and describe the nature of the work supervised.

   _____

   _____

   _____

REFERENCES

Assessment of Public Health Laboratory Management Practices. Atlanta: National Communicable Disease Center.

This document is a copy of an extensive 86-page questionnaire designed to assess the actual management practices of state laboratory directors. Section 1 contains 83 specific management tasks about which the same series of questions are asked. Section 2 then asks respondents to check the 10 most critical tasks.

Shettel, H., Hughes, R. S., and Johnson, V. F: *The Occupational Health Nurse and Employer Mental Health Final Report.* Pittsburgh, Pa.: American Institutes for Research, 1971, 75 pages plus appendices.

After extensive pilot testing a 13-page questionnaire was distributed to 14,700 occupational nurses. The instrument was designed to ascertain the nature and extent of mental health problems, as well as to ascertain nurse attitudes toward mental health problems and their present ability to cope with such problems. Data were used to design a course to enable occupational nurses to work more effectively with mental health problems.

Yankauer, A., Connelly, J., and Feldman, J.: A survey of allied health worker utilization in pediatric practices in Massachusetts and in the United States. *Pediatrics 42*: 733-42, 1968.

Report on research study in which data was collected by a questionnaire. The questionnaire was mailed to all fellows of the American Academy of Pediatrics in Massachusetts and to a 2% random sample of fellows in all other states. It inquired about current use of allied health professionals in actual practice and opinions on the subject. Almost 90% of the questionnaires were returned. The article presents the results in detail.

CRITICAL INCIDENT TECHNIQUE

DESCRIPTION

The **critical incident technique** involves collecting first-hand reports of **effective** and **ineffective** behaviors that have been observed as part of actual practice within a specified role.

An **incident** is defined as any occurrence of observable human activity that is a separate unit of experience, sufficiently complete in itself to permit inferences to be made about the person performing the act.

To be **critical**, an incident must demonstrate that the act made a difference between success and failure in carrying out an important aspect of the designated activity.

Selected observers are usually asked to recall and write down one or more incidents in which a practitioner of the role being studied **did** something that led to or caused a noticeably positive effect relative to the responsibility being discharged. And, vice versa, to recall specific situations in which some **act** led to a noticeably detrimental effect relative to what was intended.

Reports are usually obtained from observers who are familiar with many incidents of the activity. For most positions, the best observers are supervisors whose role it is to see that the particular job is done. However, in many cases, subordinates or "consumers" of the service can contribute useful observations.

ADVANTAGES

- Many incidents can be collected relatively quickly.

- Particularly good when the tasks and procedures within given responsibilities are ambiguous, highly variant, or otherwise difficult to analyze.

- The incidents themselves serve as an excellent source of examples, case studies, role plays, or problems that can be used during the course itself.

LIMITATIONS

- There is some question as to whether or not the collection of critical incidents will identify **all** the critical requirements of the position.

- Analysis of the data is cumbersome, as incidents are written in many styles with varying degrees of detail.

- Classification schemes must be developed intuitively from the actual incidents that are collected.

EXAMPLES   The next three pages contain examples of

(a) a blank form asking for an **effective** incident (ineffective or negative blanks are identical except for the substitutions of the word "ineffective" whenever "effective" appears),

(b) actual incidents collected, both effective and ineffective, and

(c) some of the categories developed in the analysis of one critical incident study.

EXAMPLE OF A
POSITIVE
CRITICAL
INCIDENT
BLANK

EFFECTIVE

From your experience, think of the **most recent situation** in which you observed an Orthopedic Surgeon do something that impressed you as an outstanding example of effective professional performance.

1. What was the situation? (Briefly describe relevant aspects of the background to the incident.)

2. How experienced was the physician involved? (Year of residency, years of post-resident practice, Board certified, etc.)

3. Exactly what did the Orthopedic Surgeon do? (Continue on other side of page, if necessary.)

4. Why was this action particularly effective; what less effective behavior might be expected in a situation like this?

Source. J. M. Blum and R. Fitzpatric, *Critical Performance Requirements for Orthopedic Surgery, Part I: Method.* Pittsburgh, Pa; American Institutes for Research, 1965.

EXAMPLES OF CRITICAL INCIDENTS

The incidents described below were collected by Blum and Fitzpatrick while developing a measure of student performance in **comprehensive medicine**. These incidents were categorized under the performance area:

Making health care accessible—The physician should take steps to bring medical care within the reach and financial means of his patient.

Effective Incident

Situation: Mother called student and described her child's illness.

Action: Student decided to make a home visit with his preceptor because mother did not have immediate transportation.

Why effective: Student was aware of other than strict medical factors in making his decision.

Less effective: A less effective student might have insisted that the mother come to the office or hospital with the child.

Ineffective Incident

Situation: Patient is a 31-year-old male with cerebral palsy referred to Neurology Clinic after extensive treatment in radiotherapy for cancer of the larynx. He is fiercely independent, lives alone, and manages all daily activities himself, has income of $81 per month.

Action: After examination in Neurology Clinic, patient was instructed by student to return in two weeks in early A.M. for X rays and lab work and to see neurologist at 1 P.M. The patient protested that he lived "too far away to be in for a morning appointment," "can't afford it," (he hired neighbor to bring him to clinic at cost of $25) and "don't see that it's necessary." The student neglected to make special arrangements for transportation.

Why ineffective: The student should have contacted other departments and community agencies to secure services, e.g., transportation, needed by the patient.

EXAMPLE OF CATEGORIES DEVELOPED FROM A CRITICAL INCIDENT STUDY

THE PHYSICIAN*

History	All actions that pertain to eliciting, recording, verifying, interpreting complete history.
Physical examination	Performing complete physical examination; acts of noting, discovering, finding; techniques.
Use of instruments	Use of instruments for examining patient: ophthalmoscope, otoscope, stethoscope, etc.
Laboratory	Use of laboratory, as in ordering tests, and interpreting results; reliance; selectivity.
X ray	Use of radiologic techniques; interpretation or use of interpretations of X rays.
Arriving at diagnosis	Making or considering diagnosis; differential diagnosis; awareness or recognition of causes, conditions, diagnoses.
Arriving at plan of treatment	Deciding on a plan of treatment, for example, to use drugs, surgery, dialysis, etc.
Review of problem	Review of records; reevaluation, reexaminations, reinvestigation; discussing problem with patient's previous physicians.
Patient education	Instructing, explaining; preparing patients. Purpose is increased patient knowledge and understanding of condition or regimen.
Psychological support	Reassuring; alleviating concern; expressing interest in patient, family. Goal is improved emotional state.
Use of community resources	Use of special agencies, community health facilities, family services, child guidance, visiting nurse association, etc.
Drugs, biological, electrolytes, fluids	Administering; prescribing; knowledge of dose; awareness of side effects.

*Source. Adapted from P. J. Sanazaro and J. W. Williamson, A classification of physician performance in internal medicine. *Journal of Medical Education. 43*: 389-397, 1968.

REFERENCES

Blum, J. M. and Fitzpatrick, R.: *Critical Performance Requirements for Orthopedic Surgery*. Pittsburgh, Pa.: American Institutes for Research, 1965. (AIR-E6-2/65-TR)

Two-part report of an extensive study of the performance of orthopedic surgeons. Part I contains an explanation of the method and plan of data collection. Part II gives behavioral descriptions of the various categories of competence, and in most cases, actual examples of both effective and ineffective performance drawn from the incident pool.

Blum, J. M. and Fitzpatrick, R.: *The Development of a Measure of Student Performance in Comprehensive Medicine*. Pittsburgh, Pa.: American Institutes for Research, 1965. (AIR-E2-4/65-TR)

Report of a study conducted in conjunction with the American Association of Medical Colleges to define comprehensive medicine empirically, distinguish comprehensive medical training from more traditional approaches, and develop instruments on the basis of empirically derived criteria by which 4th-year medical students could be evaluated. About 600 critical incidents were collected and classified, and a series of checklists were designed for evaluation purposes.

Fivars, G. and Gosnell, D.: Nursing Evaluation: *The Problem and the Process—The Critical Incident Technique*. New York: The MacMillan Company, 227 pages, 1966.

Describes how to collect critical incidents for evaluating nursing behavior, establishing institutional objectives, developing curriculum and course content consistent with these objectives, and selecting learning experiences designed to meet educational needs. Chapter 2 contains an excellent general description of how to use the critical incident technique.

Flanagan, J. C.: The critical incident technique. *Psychological Bulletin. 51:* 327-358, 1954.

One of the first attempts to describe the scope of the critical incident technique. Includes background, developmental research, and procedures for designing critical incident data collection and for analyzing the data collected.

Sanazaro, P. J. and Williamson, J. W.: A classification of physician performance in internal medicine. *Journal of Medical Education. 43:* 389-397, 1968.

Report of the analysis of 2589 critical incidents related to performance of specialists in internal medicine. The incidents were classified according to reported effects on patients.

Sanazaro, P. J. and Williamson, J. W.: Physician performance and its effects on patients: A classification based on reports by internists, surgeons, pediatricians, and obstetricians. *Medical Care.* *8*: 299-308, 1970.

Over 9100 reports of patient care incidents were obtained from over 2300 practicing specialists in internal medicine, surgery, pediatrics, and obstetrics-gynecology. These reported critical physician actions and patient results were inductively classified. These classifications contributed to the development of more systematic criteria of effective and ineffective physician performance.

THE LOG DIARY

DESCRIPTION

The **log diary** technique involves having practitioners keep track of their own daily professional activities. Usually respondents describe their professional activities at short intervals (every half hour, every hour) or immediately after each professional activity on randomly selected days.

Some log diary recording forms (see example below) call for factual details under headings such as patient care, clinical problems, clinical tests, research activity, and teaching activity. The respondent is given explicit directions on how to use the forms, usually with a completed example. The forms are designed so as to allow the respondent to supply information quickly and clearly. The log diary is often used in conjunction with a questionnaire or an interview.

ADVANTAGES

- Gives reliable information on health professional activity comparable to that obtained by direct observation.

- Allows the investigator to compare estimates of time spent with actual performance records.

- Less expensive than direct observation.

LIMITATIONS

- Respondents may make mistakes in interpreting log diary instructions and thus make mistakes in filling out the form.

- Respondents may fill out the form inaccurately because they have not kept accurate accounts of activities and time spent.

- Respondent may fill out the form in a cursory manner because they consider the task an infringement on privacy or an unnecessary burden.

EXAMPLE

Dr. Osler Peterson of the Harvard Medical School is using the log diary format to study surgical services in the United States. This study, sponsored by the American College of Surgeons and the American Surgical Association, has involved a sample of 10,000 surgeons in the United States. Respondents have been asked to fill out a questionnaire that includes a log diary. Dr. Peterson validated the questionnaire by having 150 U. S. medical students observe surgeon activity. Data from the study will be used to answer questions about surgical practice and surgical training.

EXAMPLE OF A LOG DIARY

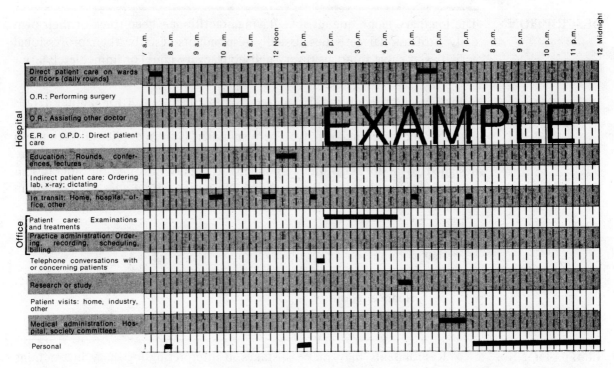

6.04

This item seeks a description of the patients you saw, treated, or advised during your assigned day which you described on the Log Diary. Please check the boxes appropriate to each patient. If an operative procedure was involved, please write it in the provided column.

		Type of Patient			Place of Care					Type of Care				
		One or Two			Check One					One or Two				
For Office Use Only		Referred By Physician	Old Patient	New Patient	Operating Room	Hospital Ward	Emergency/ OPD	Office	Patient Home or Other	Operation	Pre— or Postoperative Care	Nonsurgical Problem	Consultation	Principal Operative Procedure
	Patient number	1	2	3	1	2	3	4	5	1	2	3	4	
1 Nervous system 83	1													
2 Endocrine 28	2													
3 Eye 314	3													

Source. Osler Peterson, et al: Study on Surgical Services for the United States, American College of Surgeons, American Surgical Association, in press.

REFERENCES   Mendenhall, R. C. and Abrahamson, S.: The practical utility of log-diaries in describing physician activities. *Proceedings 12th Annual Conference on Research in Medical Education*, pp. 7-11, November 1973.

The authors analyzed 364 log diaries of cardiologists in order to obtain information on types of patients treated, methods employed in patient treatment, amount of time spent on professionally related activity, the degree to which the particular practice involved research and teaching and allocation of physician time to the range of professionally related activities.

Colten, T., Feldman, C. et al. The faculty function study at the Harvard Medical School (in press).

The authors used a log diary entitled "Activity Questionnaire" in order to determine what activities Harvard Medical School faculty pursued in the area of research teaching and service.

Peterson, O. et al. Study on surgical services for the United States. American College of Surgeons, American Surgical Association (in press).

Dr. Peterson and his colleagues are using a questionnaire supplemented by a log diary to describe surgeon performance in the U.S. Questionnaires have been distributed to a sample of 10,000 surgeons. Data is presently being collected and analyzed.

CHECKLIST

DESCRIPTION

A checklist is a closed-ended questionnaire involving a list of task statements that describe elements of the job. Large numbers of individuals who are actually performing in the position are asked to check those tasks they do in their work. Sometimes respondents are also asked to indicate additional information about the tasks they check, such as amount of time spent doing it, criticality to the job, etc.

ADVANTAGES

- Permits recognition of job tasks rather than recall. Recalling tasks is considerably less dependable but essential to many of the other methods.

- Relatively inexpensive way of collecting large amounts of data.

- Responses are easily adaptable to machine tabulation and application of pertinent statistical techniques including correlation, cluster analysis, and pattern analysis.

- Easy to identify and compare the relative importance of different tasks by obtaining time and criticality estimates for each task performed.

LIMITATIONS

- Difficult to write task statements to which an unequivocal response can be given.

- Task statements are not always mutually exclusive, and their scope depends on the judgment of the checklist constructor.

- The tedium of completing a lengthy checklist, even though structured, may result in disinterest and low motivation and, consequently, in unreliable results.

EXAMPLE OF A CHECKLIST

JOB INVENTORY *(Duty–Task List)* PAGE 5 OF 20 PAGES		RATING SCALE	RATING SCALE
LISTED BELOW ARE A DUTY AND THE TASKS WHICH IT INCLUDES. CHECK ALL TASKS WHICH YOU PERFORM. ADD ANY TASK YOU DO WHICH ARE NOT LISTED, THEN RATE THE TASK YOU HAVE CHECKED		1. very much below average 2. much below average 3. below average 4. slightly below average 5. above average 6. slightly above average 7. about average 8. much above average 9. very much above average	1. very much below average 2. much below average 3. below average 4. slightly below average 5. above average 6. slightly above average 7. about average 8. much above average 9. very much above average
DUTY: C: SUPERVISING	CHECK √ IF		
TASKS INCLUDED IN ABOVE DUTY	DONE	Importance	Time Spent
1. Advise subordinates in solving technical maintenance problems			
2. Assign workloads to personnel			
3. Counsel personnel concerning personal problems			
4. Counsel subordinates on performance or professional development			
5. Supervise corrective action concerning inspection reports			
6. Supervise maintenance inspections			
7. Supervise maintenance of aircraft carrying VIP personnel			
8. Supervise maintenance of technical publications and directives			
9. Supervise maintenance supervisors in conducting OJT programs			
10. Supervise security procedures			
11. Supervi　　　　　　　　orts on equipment			
12.			

Notice the two rating scales provided.

Source. J. R. Cragun and E. J. McCormick: *Job Inventory Information.* Lackland Air Force Base, Texas: Personnel Research Laboratory, 1967 (PRL-TR-67-15).

REFERENCES   Christal, R. E., Chairman: *Proceedings of 19. Division of Military Psychology Symposium: Collecting, Analyzing, and Reporting Information Describing Jobs and Occupations.* 77th Annual Convention of the American Psychological Association. Lackland Air Force Base, Texas: Personnel Research Division, 1969.

A series of progress reports from several major government agencies who have developed procedures for collecting and processing great masses of job data. Particularly good is the article by Joseph Morsh, which describes the job inventory survey procedure used in the Air Force. The information obtained in this way is used to develop and validate training programs, maximize the content validity of Specialty Knowledge tests, prescribe training needs, establish career ladders, and others.

Morsh, J. E. and Archer, W. B.: *Procedural Guide for Conducting Occupational Surveys in the United States Air Force.* Lackland Air Force Base, Texas: Personnel Research Laboratory, 1967 (PRL-TR-67-11).

A booklet describing in detail the procedures for collecting, organizing, analyzing, and reporting information describing work performed by Air Force officers and airmen. Many of the procedures have applicability for any type of occupational role.

OBSERVATION INTERVIEW

DESCRIPTION

The **observation interview** is essentially the same as the individual interview except that it takes place at the *work site* while the practitioner actually performs the various activities being discussed. The interviewer observes and questions the practitioner about the tasks being done in order to obtain more complete and accurate information. Time-and-motion techniques and moving pictures are variations of this observation method. In these techniques, however, questions are not asked except to clarify the nature of the activity being timed or recorded.

ADVANTAGES

- Tends to elicit small but important details often missed in the other techniques.

- Interviewer acquires a realistic "mental picture" of the setting, conditions, and processes involved in carrying out each activity.

- Allows for probing dialogue related to unexpected activities.

- Especially good for teachers who have never performed the future roles of their students.

- Elicits valid reliable data especially if several practitioners are observed.

LIMITATIONS

- Relatively slow way to obtain data, and therefore costly in terms of man-hours.

- May interfere with the operational activities of the practitioner being observed, and in many cases involving direct patient contact, simply cannot be done.

- Requires a very alert, observant interviewer.

REFERENCES

Bergman, A. B., Dassel, S. W., and Wedgwood, R. J.: Time-motion study of practicing pediatricians. *Pediatrics 38:* 254-263, 1966.

Four practicing pediatricians were followed by an observer with a stopwatch for a total of 18 days to gain a profile of how their working days were spent. This article describes the methods used to collect and analyze the data, as well as discussing the results.

Dunn, M. A.: Development of an instrument to measure nursing performance. *Nursing Research 19:* 502-510, (Nov.-Dec.) 1970.

In order to verify a task analysis of nurse practitioners working in a clinical setting an observation technique was utilized. Behaviorally stated checklists were prepared for five nursing procedures and reviewed by a panel of experts. Weights were assigned. 35 nurse practitioners were observed and rated carrying out the procedures.

Payson, H. E. and Barchas, J. D.: A time study of medical teaching rounds. *The New England Journal of Medicine* 273: 1468-1471, 1965.

Report of observation and analysis of physician performance during medical rounds. Representative samples of medical rounds were monitored by a stopwatch on the medical services of four different hospitals. The rounds were conducted in a reasonably similar manner.

WORK PARTICIPATION

INDIVIDUAL INTERVIEW

DESCRIPTION The **work participation method** involves direct work performance by the investigator. Simple operations may be performed with little or no instruction to determine characteristics of the tasks, including timing. For more difficult operations the investigator generally works with an experienced professional who can point out and correct errors.

ADVANTAGES
- Yields highly accurate data regarding the relative difficulty of tasks, time required for doing them, criteria for completeness, and potential sources of errors.

- Provides the teacher with "real" experience from which to draw later in course design.

LIMITATIONS
- Not all activities lend themselves to this type of process.

- **Very** slow method of collecting data, and if an experienced practitioner must be present, it is expensive in terms of his time too.

INDIVIDUAL INTERVIEW

DESCRIPTION

The **individual interview** technique involves interviewing one or more professional practitioners *away from the job*. The interviewer usually asks questions from a prepared questionnaire, checklist, or format; but rephrasing, probing and additional questions invariably become a critical part of the process.

ADVANTAGES

- Allows for a flexible interaction between the interviewer and the practitioner. Thus ambiguities can be clarified and data tends to be highly reliable.

- One of the more efficient ways of collecting information, especially if the persons interviewed are knowledgeable about the professional practices not only of themselves, but also of others in related positions.

- Cost is low to moderate, and dependability of results quite good, especially if several individuals are interviewed.

LIMITATIONS

- Unless the questions are highly structured, or approximate a checklist, the responses depend to a large degree on recall.

- The method is very slow, since only one person at a time is interviewed, and complete interviews often require several hours.

- The value of results depends largely on the ability of the interviewer to focus the discussion, rephrase questions and probe into alternative activities, criteria for decisions, and explanations for unexpected answers.

- Highly impractical if information from large samples is required.

- The individuals interviewed may not be representative.

REFERENCES

Research Foundation, City University of New York: *Health Services Mobility Study*. Working Papers Nos. 10, 11; Technical Report 12. Research Foundation, C.U.N.Y., 346 Broadway, New York, N.Y. 10013: 1971-1973.

This ongoing study involving individuals working in the field of radiology, ultrasound and nuclear medicine utilized interview techniques for defining tasks. Curriculum guidelines and evaluation instruments are being derived from the analysis.

GROUP INTERVIEW*

DESCRIPTION

The **group interview** involves assembling a group of practitioners representative of the position and having each of them respond to a series of structured questions. Answers may be recorded on specially prepared forms, but advantage is gained by having the participants discuss their answers aloud.

ADVANTAGES

- Yields considerably more data than individual interviews or simple questionnaires, and yet the data is collected within a very short period of time.

- Respondents tend to become involved in this process and their interaction tends to produce highly reliable information.

- Other members of the group stimulate recall by providing anecdotes and examples.

LIMITATIONS

- Sometimes difficult to arrange, depending on location and availability of the practitioners.

- Requires considerable skill on the part of the interviewer, since he/she must lead and guide the discussion so needed information is elicited in the time available.

*Also known as using a "panel of experts."

TECHNICAL CONFERENCE

DESCRIPTION In the *technical conference technique*, a group of high-level technical or subject matter experts work together to determine the responsibilities and procedures that comprise the position under investigation. A job analyst is often required to assist in arranging the information in a usable format, but this staff person generally does *not* provide much in the way of stimuli (in contrast to the group interview situation).

ADVANTAGES
- Excellent for getting highly accurate, detailed analysis of a position.
- Group interaction and personal responsibility tend to result in thorough coverage.

LIMITATIONS
- Very expensive in terms of the time required of both the experts and the job analyst who must synthesize the information.
- Sometimes technical experts have lost touch with the basic requirements of the position and may estimate job requirements in terms of their own extensive knowledge and experience rather than that of the average competent practitioner.

REFERENCES Andrew, B. J.: A methodology for the development of examinations to assess the proficiency of health care professionals. *Proceedings of the 12th Annual Conference on Research in Medical Education:* 191-196, 1973.

A group of 20 experts reviewed existing task inventories for physician's assistants and rated tasks according to the probability that the physician's assistant would carry out that task. Tasks were also rated according to frequency of occurrence and criticality.

ANNOTATED REFERENCES

Combined Methods Performance Analysis

American Association of Medical Clinics: *Prototype Staffing Model for Evaluation and Job Design in Group Practice, Primary Care Settings.* Final Report, Contract HSM 110-71-87, 125 pages, 1973.

This ambitious study directed by Lon G. McKinnon and William F. O'Connor queried 337 member clinics. Checklists and questionnaires were utilized to study tasks in terms of: who performed each task, performance time, effect of error on patient, special equipment requirements, need for privacy, and task frequency. Data can be utilized for training requirements including structuring career ladders, evaluation of program, job design, licensing, and registration.

Clute, K. F.: *The General Practitioner: A Study of Medical Education and Practice in Ontario and Nova Scotia.* Toronto: University of Toronto Press, 566 pages, 1963.

An account of an extensive study of 86 general medical practices, with emphasis on quality and problems of medical care. Each physician filled out a lengthy questionnaire and also was observed continuously for 2 to 4 days.

Martin, M. C. and Brodt, D. E.: Task analysis for training and curriculum design. *Improving Human Performance 2:* 113-128 (Summer) 1973.

A task analysis was conducted by field interviews and observations in order to define the job of hospital corpsman. Priorities and difficulty levels were defined. Data was utilized to design training.

Peterson, O. L., Andrews, L. P., Spain, R. S., and Greenberg, B. G.: *An Analytical Study of North Carolina General Practices, 1953-1954.* Evanston, Illinois: Association of American Medical Colleges, 165 pages, 1956.

This book reports on a major research effort designed to identify those problems of general practitioners which may be solved by better education and organizational activities. Detailed questionnaires and rating criteria were used over a 3 1/2 day observation period.

Price, P. B., Taylor, E. W., Nelson, D. E. et al.: *Measurement and Predictors of Physician Performance.* Salt Lake City, Utah: Lynn Lloyd Reid Enterprises, LLR Press, 1971.

A book reporting on two decades of intermittently sustained research aimed at problems of measuring and predicting physician performance. A variety of techniques were used in the six separate studies reported.

Harless, J.: *An Ounce of Analysis (Is Worth a Pound of Objectives)*. Falls Church, Va.: Harless Educational Technologists, Inc., 79 pages, 1970.

A self-instructional programmed lesson on how to conduct a performance analysis in a training problem. Designed for use primarily by educational technologists within business and industry, but helpful to anyone who needs to analyze the causes (skill/knowledge, motivation, environment) of a given performance problem.

Mager, R. F.: *Analyzing Performance Problems or "You Really Oughta Wanna."* Belmont, Cal.: Fearon Publishers, 111 pages, 1970.

A readable book about how to solve problems that arise because someone isn't doing what someone else expects him to be doing. It explains a procedure for analyzing such problems and has particular applicability for business and industry.

A Proposal for Assisting Foreign Quarantine Programs in Determining if Differences Exist between Actual and Desired Job Performance of Foreign Quarantine Inspectors. Atlanta: National Communicable Disease Center (January 8, 1971).

Example of a detailed C.D.C. proposal for a comprehensive performance analysis of a professional position in epidemiology. Lists and describes every step to be performed.

Chapter 8

METHODS FOR PHASE 2: DESCRIBING STUDENT COMPETENCIES

Contents

PLANNING TESTS

INTRODUCTION

Chapter 8 addresses the questions that might be considered when formulating an evaluation plan:

- What are the purposes of the evaluation plan?

- What procedures should be considered for inclusion in the evaluation plan?

- How does one relate questions of validity and reliability to formulating a plan?

- How does the instructor decide among types of test instruments?

- What are the commonly used methods for grading students?

WHY BOTHER WITH EVALUATION?

In an area with as many detailed aspects as evaluation, it is easy to overlook the main purposes of evaluation as we see it: to give both the instructor and the students **feedback** on the instructional process. This major purpose of evaluation—giving feedback—speaks to an even more fundamental assumption having to do with the purpose of instruction.

In the health fields a teacher is attempting to enable students to attain mastery of certain procedures and knowledge. Feedback is introduced into the instructional process to ascertain whether or not this learning is in fact occurring.

DETERMINING EVALUATION PURPOSES AND PROCEDURES

INTRODUCTION   There are three general **purposes** of evaluation:

1. **Management** of the instructional **process** (e.g., to screen course applicants, monitor student progress, assign students to special tracks, identify problems for remediation, etc).
2. **Assessment** of the overall **success** of instruction (e.g., to measure achievement of the objectives, assign grades, etc).
3. **Improvement** of the **quality** of the instruction (e.g., to revise the course or a test instrument).

The *purposes* of an evaluation determine both the type of evaluation procedures needed and the nature of the decisions resulting from the evaluation.

EPPC   A summary of evaluation purposes and procedures is presented in the Evaluation Purposes and Procedures Chart (EPPC) on the following page. The EPPC is intended to serve as a guide in planning an overall evaluation design.

1. The first column, "Purposes of Evaluation," describes specific ways you might use evaluation data.
2. The next column, "Evaluation Procedures," indicates the types of procedures appropriate for each purpose. In some instances, a **choice** of procedures is available; in others, the use of more than one procedure is **necessary**.
3. The last column describes in general terms the decision rules or interpretations appropriate for each purpose and its associated procedure(s).

EVALUATION PURPOSES AND PROCEDURES CHART
(EPPC)

	PURPOSE OF EVALUATION	EVALUATION PROCEDURES	DECISION RULES AND INTERPRETATION
MANAGEMENT	1. To select students who need the instruction	Pretest	Low score = admit to instruction High score = bypass instruction
	2. To select students for limited course enrollment	Prerequisite test, Pretest, Attitude or Interest Tests and/or interview	Select students with high scores on prerequisite test, low scores on pretest, and/or high interest and motivation.
	3. To determine if preparatory instruction is needed	Prerequisite test keyed to preparatory instruction	Low score = give preparatory instruction High score = ready for instruction now
	4. To provide feedback to students	Progress tests, Teaching Observations, and/or Post-test(s)	Success feedback = proceed Failure feedback = diagnose problem and give remedial instruction
	5. To diagnose individual needs (for bypass or remedial instruction)	Prerequisite test, Pre-, Progress Tests, Teaching Observations and/or Student Conference	Bypass if perfect scores and student comments that "too easy or elementary." Remediation if low scores and observed trouble.
ASSESSMENT	6. To determine *if* students achieved the objectives	Posttest(s)	Low score = objectives not met High score = objectives met
	7. To determine *how much* students have learned	Pretest and Posttest	Generally, the greater the prepost difference, the greater the learning.
	8. To assign grades	Posttest; or Pre- and Post-test	Assign grades to scores; or to gain in scores.
IMPROVEMENT	9. To revise and improve instructional process	Pretest, Posttest, Progress Test, and/or Teaching Observations	Items with many errors = problems with the corresponding instruction and/or testing; look for ways to improve the instruction.
	10. To improve evaluation instruments	Instrument(s) to be investigated	Unexpected/unstable data = evaluation problem (e.g., few pretest errors, many posttest errors, unchanging error rates, etc.)

STRATEGIES FOR VALIDITY AND RELIABILITY

INTRODUCTION   The quality of an evaluation procedure is generally described in terms of its validity and reliability.

> The **validity** of a test refers to the "truth" of the measurement—the accuracy with which it measures the performance, knowledge, or attitudes it claims to measure.

> The **reliability** of a test refers to the "repeatability" of the measurement—the consistency with which it measures whatever it does measure.

Unless evaluation events represent valid and reliable measurements of the extent to which students have achieved the instructional objectives, it would be pointless to use their results for the management, assessment, or improvement of instruction.

Both validity and reliability can be assessed statistically, using data from actual administrations of the test instrument. More important at this stage, however, are the ways an instructor can design evaluation events that will constitute valid, reliable measures.

VALIDITY   To ensure validity, the conditions and performances of the evaluation events should be identical to actual conditions and performances in the real world. To the extent that the real-world activity and the corresponding evaluation event are **not** the same, the evaluation is said to "simulate" the real world. The more directly and closely one replicates the real world (i.e., the higher level of simulation), the more likely it is that the evaluation (and instruction) will be valid.

Although validity increases with level of simulation, the real-world situation itself usually cannot, and sometimes **should not**, be used for evaluation. Time, effort, danger, and lack of consistency in opportunity may make a lower level of simulation necessary.

When planning a simulation activity, an attempt should be made to replicate as many aspects of the real-world stimulus conditions and performance as possible.

For example, consider the objective, "Students will be able to diagnose, treat, and follow up cases of tuberculosis." A practical examination, though ideal from the point of view of validity, would require more time, resources, and instructor effort than is feasible. Alternatives should be considered in light of the extent to which they replicate aspects of real-world conditions.

An essay test could require the student to specify, in sequence, the procedure he would follow in treating and following up a patient with tuberculosis. Thus an essay test can assess some of the critical cognitive aspects of the real-world task. If the necessary psychomotor and interpersonal skills (such as examining the patient, taking a history, administering drugs, etc.) have already been learned by students in other courses, or can be evaluated as components apart from the overall evaluation, then the essay exam might validly assess achievement of the objective.

This is also true of a multiple-choice test. However, this type of test item may provide students with cues unavailable in the real-world situation. On the other hand, multiple-choice tests permit the instructor to pose a wider variety of real-world situations for student response than do most essay tests. In addition, the ease and objectivity of scoring a multiple-choice test compared to an essay exam might justify its use.

Whether a lower level of simulation can be used to measure validly an objective should be considered carefully. If there is any doubt regarding such a decision, the validity of the simulated method can be established statistically by correlating results obtained when using the real situation with results obtained from the simulation for the same group of students. Such a comparison is generally expressed in terms of a validity coefficient. Should computational procedures for such a statistic become necessary, consult one of the annotated references listed at the end of this unit.

RELIABILITY   Assuring reliability is somewhat more difficult than validity simply because reliability depends in part on the **constancy** of students' ability to perform the tasks presented in the test. All human beings vary from time to time in their general alertness and emotional stability, and this often affects the repeatability of their performance on any task. Nonetheless, there are several instructor-controlled factors that enhance the reliability of evaluation events.

1. Consistency in test conditions

An attempt should be made to assure that the test conditions (stimuli and resources) will be consistent from one student to another. Reliability cannot be expected if no two administrations of the test involve the same stimuli and resources.

2. Specificity and appropriateness of performance

The expected behaviors should be clearly specified and appropriate for the level of performance being assessed. Tasks that are too difficult or permit students to make widely divergent interpretations of what is expected of them are likely to yield unreliable measures.

3. Amount of real-world performance being sampled

Usually the longer the test and the more aspects of the intended performance that are sampled, the more reliable the measurement. Of course, the length of testing is constrained by the total amount of time available for instruction and evaluation.

4. Objectivity of scoring

Student performance must be scored objectively to produce reliable results. Without consistent standards of performance, applied uniformly from student to student, the resulting scores will lack reliability.

Like validity, reliability can be established statistically by a variety of methods. Most reliability coefficients are obtained by correlating two sets of scores for the same group of students. Again, should computational procedures for such a statistic become desirable, consult one of the annotated references listed at the end of this unit.

SELECTING EVALUATION TECHNIQUES

INTRODUCTION There are many different methods for observing and measuring student performance. Each is more appropriate in some types of situations than in others, and each has its advantages and disadvantages.

DIRECTORY

PRACTICAL EXAMINATIONS

DESCRIPTION

A **practical examination** is a test procedure in which the student performs the skills to be evaluated in a natural or carefully planned simulated setting. Measurements may be obtained by observing the performance itself and/or products of the performance.

EXAMPLES

1. Given a patient during a routine visit to the clinic, the student performs a physical examination.

2. Given several bacterial cultures, the student prepares slides and identifies the organisms.

3. Students demonstrate cardio-pulmonary resuscitation with a mannequin.

BEST INSTRUCTIONAL USE

- When the competency to be evaluated involves psychomotor or interpersonal behaviors.

- When conditions of performance are readily available and/or can be easily simulated.

- When behavior to be evaluated can be performed within a reasonable time period.

ADVANTAGES

- Tests ability to **apply** skills in real or simulated conditions.

- Provides opportunity to observe behaviors **related** to the main performance, such as attitudes or ability to adapt to changing conditions.

LIMITATIONS

- Difficult to standardize testing conditions because of variations

    (1) in availability of resources (such as patients exhibiting particular syndromes), and
    (2) among the resources themselves (individual differences between patients).

- Observation and scoring procedures are usually time-consuming.

- Requires time and effort to coordinate preparation of test conditions with schedules of both examiners and students.

- Sample of student behavior may be small compared to other methods.

OBSERVATIONAL REPORTS

DESCRIPTION **Observational reports** involve systematic and repeated observations of student performance over a period of time, usually in naturalistic settings. Observations are made periodically as the student conducts professional procedures in the laboratory, clinic, or ward. Often, observations are recorded on checklists or rating scales.

EXAMPLES

1. An intern is observed at different stages of patient management throughout the duration of several cases.

2. Once a day the head nurse observes each student nurse's performance for five minutes and records ratings or judgments about that performance.

3. In a dental clinic, the teacher is called over to evaluate each successive stage of a dental preparation.

BEST INSTRUCTIONAL USE

- When competency to be assessed involves a variety of stimulus conditions that cannot easily be prearranged or simulated.

- When competency involves many different components and performance takes place over a lengthy period of time.

- When competency to be evaluated is complex and involves many psychomotor and/or interpersonal behaviors.

ADVANTAGES

- Can obtain more reliable observations than with other techniques, because many behaviors are sampled over long intervals.

- Can assess professional attitudes as well as mastery of skills.

- Can pool the reports of many examiners and thereby increase the reliability of the results.

LIMITATIONS

- Presence of observer may significantly alter the behavior of the student or the patient.

- Requires extended contact with the student.

- Considerable effort is required to standardize performance criteria and report results (e.g., rating scale or checklist to be used).

ORAL EXAMINATIONS

DESCRIPTION	The **oral examination** is a testing procedure in which the student responds orally to specific questions or problems. The student may be asked to explain how he would approach a specified problem, defend his judgments, or assume a specified role in an interaction.
EXAMPLE	Given standardized case material, the student discusses with the examiner his diagnostic impressions, his reasons for them, and the next steps he would recommend for the care of the specific patient.
BEST INSTRUCTIONAL USE	• When the competency to be evaluated involves the ability to "think on one's feet" in an unpredictable interpersonal situation. • When there are few students who require testing at different times (such as in the training of interns and residents). • When flexibility in questioning needs to be maintained because the areas to be covered or the particular sequence of topics cannot be predicted beforehand.
ADVANTAGES	• Can tailor the questions to a variety of contingencies, that is, can state questions, probe in particular areas, or alter the questioning strategy. • Can assess a student's thought process or way of "thinking through" a problem. • Can take mitigating circumstances into account. • Can obtain simultaneous assessment by two or more examiners.
LIMITATIONS	• Difficult to establish standard conditions and criteria for performance. • Social interaction may influence objectivity. • Examiner may inadvertently give cues. • Time-consuming for the examiner(s).

PROJECT ASSIGNMENTS

DESCRIPTION

A **project assignment** involves giving the student a task or project to complete and then evaluating the **product(s)** of the completed performance. Products may be written, such as a paper to be turned in, or nonwritten such as a physical object or laboratory preparation.

EXAMPLES

- Research reports
- Project reports
- Case studies
- Slide preparations
- Tissue dissections
- Dental preparations

BEST INSTRUCTIONAL USES

- When the competency to be evaluated involved steps that are performed over a period of time and culminate in an observable product.

- When primarily interested in the product rather than the means of creating the product.

- When features of the product reflect the performance to be evaluated.

ADVANTAGES

- Can be used to evaluate complex behaviors that require considerable time to perform and are otherwise difficult to observe directly.

- The product, being static, is available for careful assessment, over time.

- Assesses the ability to work independently.

- Reflects ability to collect and synthesize real-world data.

LIMITATIONS

- Indirect measurement of real-world performance since product is observed.

- Sometimes difficult to prevent cheating, plagiarism, etc.

- Cannot assess the performance process itself, such as amount of outside assistance received or amount of time and effort consumed in producing product.

- Developing standards for judging the quality of student product(s) may be difficult, and applying these standards consistently may be time-consuming.

ESSAY EXAMINATIONS

DESCRIPTION	An **essay examination** is a test procedure in which the student responds in written form to specific problems or questions.
EXAMPLE 1	1. Given a letter from a community group requesting advice on how to set up a particular type of community health service, the student drafts a reply.
	2. Given an X ray and supplementary information, the intern reconstructs the history that led to the findings and outlines and justifies his recommendations for patient management.
	3. Given a copy of a hospital chart, the student writes a discharge letter to the patient's family physician.
BEST INSTRUCTIONAL USES	• When assessing analytic abilities and skill in written expression.
	• When more convenient to spend time scoring an examination than constructing it.
	• When group to be tested is small.
	• In early stages of developing an assessment instrument, in order to gather data for later construction of an "objective" test (e.g., to collect common misconceptions to serve as distractors in multiple-choice items).
ADVANTAGES	• Can assess a student's ability to recall information, organize ideas, and express them effectively in his/her words.
	• Easier to prepare essay questions than other types of items.
LIMITATIONS	• Difficult to establish objective scoring standards.
	• May discriminate against students with poor verbal abilities.
	• Time-consuming to score and to provide adequate feedback to students.

OBJECTIVE EXAMINATIONS

DESCRIPTION

An **objective examination** is a test procedure in which the scoring of responses does not depend on the subjective judgment of the examiner as in other forms of testing. This includes both **selection** items (multiple-choice, true-false, matching, ranking-in-order) and **production** items (fill-in-the blanks, etc). The question or problem posed is usually written, but visual or auditory materials can be used as part of the stimulus.

EXAMPLES

1. Given a partially filled-in table, the student completes the table.

2. Given a tape-recording of heart sounds, the student answers a series of multiple-choice questions regarding what he hears.

3. Given a case description of a patient and a series of suggested treatments, the student selects the most likely result from a set of six possible results.

BEST INSTRUCTIONAL USES

- When the group of students to be tested is large.

- When a systematic sampling of students' knowledge must be obtained, since a large area of knowledge must be assessed in a short period of time.

- When there is more pressure for rapid reporting of scores than for rapid test preparation.

- When a reliable instrument that can produce standardized results for a large population is needed.

- When objectives involve abilities such as identifying relevant aspects of problems, discriminating between various symptoms or characteristics, or applying principles to a variety of new situations.

ADVANTAGES

- Scoring is easy, unambiguous, and less time-consuming than for any other method of evaluation.

- Can sample variety of facts and intellectual processes in a comparatively short period of time.

- Easy to give complete feedback to students.

- Objectivity of scoring permits use of test statistics and item analysis for improving test and pinpointing problems in the instruction.

LIMITATIONS

- Construction is time-consuming if ambiguous questions are to be avoided.

- Correct answers may be achieved by guessing (especially if number of alternatives is limited as in true-false items).

- May discriminate against poor readers, since a great deal of critical reading is required of students.
- Presence of correct alternatives may prompt response.
- Production items (fill-in-the-blanks) can involve difficulty in determining acceptable alternate responses.

ATTITUDINAL MEASURES

INTRODUCTION There are two main occasions on which a teacher in the health fields may be concerned with measuring attitudes:

(a) Having attempted to influence student attitudes using one or more of the methods described in Chapter 9, the instructor may be interested in determining the effectiveness of the teaching strategy.

(b) During or on completion of a course, the instructor may wish to ascertain students' attitudes toward the instruction itself for purposes of identifying areas needing improvement.

It must be emphasized that attitudes are difficult to specify in precise terms and, therefore, to measure definitively. The study of attitudes and their measurement is a discipline in its own right, and it is beyond the scope of this book to deal comprehensively with the subject.

DESCRIPTION Attitudes in relation to instructional situations can be measured either through paper-and-pencil tests or by instructor observations and ratings of student performance, especially in conjunction with tests of student competencies at higher levels of simulation (e.g., posttests). The former will be referred to here as **attitude tests**, the latter as **behavior ratings**.

ATTITUDE TESTS Two well-known types of attitude tests are those developed by Thurstone and Likert.

- The **Thurstone method** involves collecting numerous statements that describe a variety of possible beliefs about a specific attitude object. These statements are then rank-ordered by a panel of experts. Only those statements are retained on which consensus is reached, and the result is a series of statements that presumably represent equidistant positions along a continuum ranging from highly positive to highly negative attitudes. The respondent indicates those statements that correspond to her/his own position.

- **Likert scales** are somewhat more simple to construct. A statement of an attitude is accompanied by a scale from one to five (or seven) representing the range from high agreement to high disagreement with the statement. The respondent then indicates her/his position on this scale.

BEHAVIOR RATINGS **Behavior ratings** require the development of instruments to help the instructor observe and describe a given performance. Typically a set of behavior descriptions are listed, all or some of which are assumed to be indicative of a given attitude. Given a structured performance situation, such as a posttest or other high level of simulation, the observer records the frequency of the behaviors listed during specified time samples and/or gives a summary rating at the end of the observation period.

EXAMPLES	1. A portion of a Likert-type attitude test is shown on page C-46. 2. One scale from a behavior rating instrument is shown on page C-47.

BEST INSTRUCTIONAL USES

- Attitude tests are best used for determining students' attitudes toward:
  - (a) various issues associated with the professional responsibilities to which the course objectives are directed, and
  - (b) the course itself.
- Behavior ratings are best used for evaluating attitudinal aspects of student terminal competencies (e.g., as the basic instrument for or supplements to posttests that involve actual or simulated practical examinations).

ADVANTAGES

- Attitude tests are easy to administer and score (although time-consuming to develop properly).
- Behavior ratings may give a more valid picture of the individual's attitude toward the professional responsibilities.

LIMITATIONS

- Attitude tests are easy for students to fake, as the "right answers" may often be obvious within the context of the test.
- Behavior ratings are time-consuming to develop and administer and may require training in the use of the instrument.
- It may be difficult to design situations for behavior ratings within which enough relevant incidents of the behavior in question can occur.

EXHIBIT 3-26

THE CUSTODIAL MENTAL ILLNESS
IDEOLOGY (CMI) SCALE

This is part of a larger study by the Russell Sage Foundation. We are interested in the various ways of thinking about mental illness and some related social problems. We are trying to get answers from various groups in different parts of the country. The groups will include the general public as well as those of you who have had direct experience with hospitalized patients, i.e., nurses, attendants, and doctors.

The best answer to each statement below is your *personal opinion*. We have tried to cover many different points of view. You may find yourself agreeing strongly with some of the statements, disagreeing just as strongly with others.

Mark each statement in the left margin according to how much you agree or disagree with it. *Please mark every one.* Write in +1, +2, +3, or –1, –2, –3, depending on how you feel in each case.

+1 I AGREE A LITTLE	–1 I DISAGREE A LITTLE
+2 I AGREE PRETTY MUCH	–2 I DISAGREE PRETTY MUCH
+3 I AGREE VERY MUCH	–3 I DISAGREE VERY MUCH

 1 Only persons with considerable psychiatric training should be allowed to form close relationships with patients.

 2 It is best to prevent the more disturbed patients from mixing with those who are less sick.

 3 As soon as a person shows signs of mental disturbance he should be hospitalized.

*4 Mental illness is an illness like any other.

 5 Close association with mentally ill people is liable to make even a normal person break down.

 6 We can make some improvements, but by and large the conditions of mental hospital wards are about as good as can be considering the type of disturbed patient living there.

 7 We should be sympathetic with mental patients, but we cannot expect to understand their odd behavior.

 8 One of the main causes of mental illness is lack of moral strength.

*9 When a patient is discharged from a hospital, he can be expected to carry out his responsibilities as a citizen.

10 Abnormal people are ruled by their emotions; normal people by their reason.

11 A mental patient is in no position to make decisions about even everyday living problems.

*12 Patients are often kept in the hospital long after they are well enough to get along in the community.

13 There is nothing about mentally ill people that makes it easy to tell them from normal people.

*Items marked with an asterisk are "humanistic"; others are "custodial."

Source. M. E. Shaw and J. M. Wright: *Scales for the Measurement of Attitudes.* New York: McGraw-Hill, 1967, p. 110.
[Adapted from Gilbert, Doris C., and Levinson, D. J.: " 'Custodialism' and 'Humanism' in Mental Hospital Structure and in Staff Ideology." Pp. 20-35 in Greenblatt, M., Levinson, D., and Williams, R. (Eds.): *The Patient and the Mental Hospital.* New York: The Free Press (Macmillan Co.), 1957.]

The Medical Instruction Observation Record, developed to assess medical instruction, has seven major dimensions (attitude to individual differences, sensitivity to physical setting, attitude to students and patients, use of instructional materials, reaction to students' needs, use of teaching methods and use of "challenge." Actually, a rating schedule rather than a category system, each of the scales is divided into 22 points, with detailed behaviorally specified examples being cited every five points along the scale. This work is of particular interest because of its efforts to translate evidence of "attitudes" into behaviorally specified dimensions and because of its focus on the affective dimensions of medical education and away from effects of traditionally acknowledged pressage variables such as knowledge in subject matter, professional experience, professional preparation or amount of teaching experience.

CATEGORIES FOR
MEDICAL INSTRUCTION OBSERVATION RECORD (MIOR)

Hilliard Jason

ATTITUDE TO DIFFERENCE   Scale I

A
B   Rejects questions that reflect poor understanding on the part of the student. Insults a student who
C   disagrees with his own opinions.
D
E

F
G   Indicates by innuendo and gesture that differences are not desirable. Without directly saying so, makes it
H   clear to the students that disagreement with him is encouraged.
I

J
K
L
M   Without showing much pleasure or displeasure, deals patiently with disagreements, and with differences
N   in degrees of understanding.
O
P

Q
R   Actively encourages group disagreement and discussion. Reacts to criticism with interest and
S   understanding. Encourages individuals to express their points of view.
T

X   Insufficient evidence.

Y   Inappropriate for this session.

COMMENTS AND ANECDOTAL EVIDENCE:

Source. A. Simon, and E. Boyer: *Mirrors for Behavior II*, Vol. B. Philadelphia: Research for Better Schools Inc., 1970.

GRADING STUDENTS

INTRODUCTION If evaluation has a bad reputation, it is due to the inequities that students of all educational levels attribute to the grading systems which have been imposed on their learning. A preliminary consideration of norm-referenced and criterion-referenced grading systems will clarify some of the issues involved and perhaps suggest options to the instructor that he has not previously considered.

DIRECTORY

NORM-REFERENCED GRADING SYSTEMS

DESCRIPTION

Norm-referenced grading systems are designed to measure an individual's performance in comparison with the performance of a group of students, usually one's classmates. The comparison group, however, may be a larger group, that is, all medical students in New York State or all orthopedic residents in the United States. To assign norm-referenced grades, the instructor arranges a distribution of or rank-orders the students according to their performance (i.e., scores) on the test or set of tests and then decides what proportion of students should receive an A, B, C, D, or E or equivalent.

The normal curve may be used to make the determination of how many students to include in each category. If the normal curve is used, the distribution of grades would approximate that shown below:

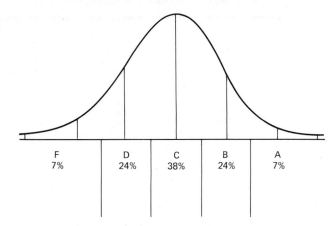

F	D	C	B	A
7%	24%	38%	24%	7%

Normal curve with a typical distribution of grades.

Source. N. E. Gronlund: *Improving Marking and Reporting in Classroom Instruction.* New York: Macmillan, 1974.

The normal curve, however, is just one method of assigning norm-referenced grades. The instructor might, for example, decide to use the following schema or an adaptation thereof:

A	10-20%
B	20-30%
C	40-50%
D	10-20%
E	0-10

Instructors decide what proportion of students should receive each grade on the basis of personal experience with student groups or on the grading practices within his institution.

| **BEST INSTRUCTIONAL USE** | • When test score distributions approximate the normal curve. |
| | • When the instructor wishes to spread student scores on a continuum for purposes of making administrative decisions, that is, providing remediation, or selecting students for an honors seminar, etc. |

| **ADVANTAGES** | • Facilitates comparison among individuals. |
| | • Conforms with prevailing practices in most educational situations. |

| **LIMITATIONS** | • Most actual distributions of student scores do not approximate a normal curve or expected distribution. |
| | • The comparative status of students may or may not be a valid indication of the overall level of mastery attained (e.g., just what does an "A" or a "C" mean with respect to demonstrated accomplishment of student terminal competencies?) |

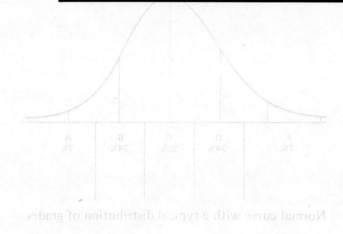

Normal curve with a typical distribution of grades

Source: N. E. Gronlund, *Improving Marking and Reporting in Classroom Instruction*, New York: Macmillan, 1974.

The normal curve, however, is just one method of assigning norm-referenced grades. The instructor might, for example, decide to use the following schema or an adaptation thereof:

A   10-20%
B   20-30%
C   40-50%
D   10-20%
E   0-10

Instructors decide what proportion of students should receive each grade on the basis of personal experience with student groups or on the grading practices within his institution.

CRITERION-REFERENCED GRADING SYSTEMS

DESCRIPTION

Criterion-referenced tests are designed to evaluate student achievement in relation to previously specified performance standards. The objective of such tests is to determine whether the student has attained mastery of a given procedure, not comparison of students with one another. The philosophy of criterion-referenced tests is thus very different from that used in norm-referenced testing.

It is possible using a system of criterion-referenced tests to have all students receive an A. In fact, if the instructional system has been designed to facilitate achievement of the objectives—demonstrated attainment of student terminal competencies—it could be expected that all or nearly all of the students would do very well on the posttest.

Developing a criterion-referenced test involves the procedures described in this book: the instructor

    (a) specifies mastery,

    (b) decides the highest level of simulation that can be attained in the classroom,

    (c) defines conditions and performance for each classroom objective,

    (d) decides on the criterion that will be applied to determine if the learner has achieved the student terminal competency, and

    (e) constructs tests/instruments that reflect the above analysis. Behavior ratings may be necessary tools.

BEST INSTRUCTIONAL USE

- When a model for systematic course design has been applied.

- When performance criteria are communicated to students at the onset of instruction so they can work toward mastery of each skill.

ADVANTAGES

- Compares each student's performance with a rationally derived criterion rather than with the varying achievement of a comparison group.

LIMITATIONS

- Standard mathematical calculations for test reliability and item analysis only partially apply.

- Hard to define criteria for mastery of any given procedure because of lack of agreement among experts.

- Because high levels of simulation are often involved, test administration may be time-consuming and costly.

- Ensuring adequate reliability is time-consuming and may require training of those who apply the criteria.

REFERENCES

Bloom, B. S., Hastings, S. T., and Madaus, A. F.: *Handbook on Formative and Summative Evaluation of Student Learning.* New York: McGraw Hill, 1971.

An excellent text on the design of cognitive and affective tests. Stresses the need to evaluate at high level of simulation. Many examples.

Ebel, Robert L.: *Essentials of Educational Measurement.* Englewood Cliffs, N.J.: Prentice-Hall, Inc., 1972.

A relatively short book, very readable, but packed with a great deal of well-organized information and suggestions. Probably the best available short text on measurement and test construction. (This book is the second edition of a book formerly titled Measuring Educational Achievement, *1965.)*

Furst, Edward J.: *Constructing Evaluation Instruments.* New York: Longmans, Green, 1958.

Rich with practical examples of items, objectives, and ways of organizing tests.

Gronlund, N. E.: *Improving Marking and Reporting in Classroom Instruction.* New York, Macmillan, 1974.

A brief readable book with useful chapters in assigning norm-referenced letter grades and on criterion-referenced marking and reporting.

Mager, R. F.: *Measuring Instructional Intent or Gota Match?* Belmont, California: Fearon, 1973.

An excellent book enabling the reader to specify conditions and performance of mastery as a basis for constructing test instruments.

Miller, Richard I.: *Evaluating Faculty Performance.* San Francisco: Jossey-Bass, 1972.

This book concentrates on faculty self-evaluation. It includes many practical suggestions, including questionnaires for student, faculty, and administration use.

Payne, David A. *The Specification and Measurement of Learning Outcomes.* Waltham, Mass.: Blaisdell, 1968.

An excellent brief text.

Popham, J. (Ed.): *Criterion-Referenced Measurement: An Introduction.* Englewood Cliffs, N. J.: Educational Technology Publications, 1971.

A compilation of papers by leaders in the field including an excellent paper by Popham discussing methods for analyzing criterion-referenced tests.

Shaw, M. E. and Wright, J. M.: *Scales for the Measurement of Attitudes.* New York: McGraw Hill, 1967.

A useful compendium of paper-and-pencil attitude tests including attitudinal tests concerned with health-related issues, practices, and institutions. Attitude tests on other social science topics are included. Information on scoring as well as reliability and validity of instruments is included.

Simon, A. and Boyer, E. G.: *Mirrors for Behavior II* , Vols. A and B. 1700 Market Street, Philadelphia, Pa.: Research for Better Schools, Inc., 1970.

An excellent collection of behavior rating instruments including a number of instruments useful for teacher preparation in the health fields. A good summary of the utility and potential of behavior ratings is included.

Thorndike, Robert L. (ed.): *Educational Measurement.* (2nd ed.) Washington: American Council on Education, 1971.

This is the standard handbook on educational measurement. This volume discusses all aspects of test construction, but at a level useful primarily to individuals with specialized interest and training in evaluation. It contains an excellent chapter on the evaluation of performance and products.

Webb, Eugene J., et al. *Unobtrusive Measures: Nonreactive Research in the Social Sciences.* Chicago: Rand-McNally, 1966.

Not on test construction in the usual sense of the word, but covers a variety of measures, many of which are rarely used, but highly applicable to medical and public health problems.

Chapter 9

METHODS FOR PHASE 3: PLANNING STUDENT LEARNING

Contents

(Contents, continued)

METHODS FOR DEVELOPING ATTITUDES IN THE CLASSROOM

INTRODUCTION The successful instructor is inevitably concerned with his student's attitudes. The first and most important reason is that a positive attitude toward learning greatly facilitates the learning process. Students who want to learn do so faster than those who have a negative attitude about learning. Second, developing attitudes in the students about their work may be one of the instructor's main teaching objectives. The instructor may decide that his students, to be successful health care workers after graduation, must acquire not only professional skills and knowledge but also certain attitudes about their work. Nurses, physicians, social workers, dentists, and the like will not achieve their full working potential without a positive regard for themselves, their work, and their patients. Thus, for both of these reasons, the instructor must prepare himself to work with attitudes in the classroom.

DIRECTORY

TRANSMITTING INFORMATION

INTRODUCTION   People sometimes adopt certain attitudes on the basis of misinformation or because they have inadequate information on the issue in question. One way to develop a positive attitude or to change a negative one is to provide factual information supporting the new viewpoint.

DESCRIPTION   The instructor merely furnishes information thought to be conducive to changing student attitudes in the desired direction.

ADVANTAGES
- Not laborious or time-consuming for the instructor.
- May be used in conjunction with other methods for shaping attitudes.

LIMITATIONS   Usually attitudes are emotionally based, at least in part, and therefore students may need active, emotional-motivational experiences before they develop significant new attitudes or change old ones. Merely reading a book, listening to a lecture, or watching television may not be effective. It has been found, for example, that people tend to watch only those programs and to read only those newspapers that support their existing attitudes. The adoption of a new attitude as a result of mass communication alone usually occurs only in a small minority of cases. Providing new information may be helpful but further effort is usually necessary.

EXAMPLE 1   Some years ago university psychologists attempted to induce students to adopt a home program of dental hygiene. In some instances the students were merely presented with information on dental care. In other instances they were shown vivid illustrations of the mouth and tooth diseases that can result when proper dental care is neglected. Results of this study indicated that information, by itself, was more effective in changing attitudes and behavior than were those presentations that aroused a high degree of fear among the students. Sometimes, the mere presentation of information can be effective; the use of an emotional appeal, such as fear, is not necessarily more effective.

EXAMPLE 2   An urban medical student, trained in the traditional manner, may know very little about folk medicine and home remedies. Furthermore, he may have adopted a negative attitude toward these practices because other "educated" people seem to regard them negatively. When exposed to information about the curative results of these practices in certain subcultures, he may alter his outlook. His negative attitude may change to acceptance or even to support in appropriate instances.

REFERENCES   Hovland, C. I. and Weiss, W.: The influence of source credibility on communication effectiveness. *Public Opinion Quarterly. 15:* 635-650, 1951.

This extensive research program emphasizes what many writers have suspected: the single most important factor in determining whether people accept or reject information is their opinion of the person who communicates it. In the classroom, therefore, the students' opinions of their teacher are most important in determining whether they believe the information he presents to them.

Janis, I. L. and Feshbach, S.: Effects of fear-arousing communications. *Journal of Abnormal and Social Psychology. 48:* 78-92, 1953.

These are the classic studies in which attempts were made to induce high school students to adopt a program of dental hygiene. It was found that an appeal based strictly on accurate dental information and care of the teeth was superior to one in which fear also was invoked in the audience. Potential changes in attitude and behavior seemed to have been suppressed when the students were made highly anxious by strong, fear-arousing communications.

PROVIDING A MODEL

DESCRIPTION

A model is something to be copied. It is intended to be close to the perfect or ideal form of something, or at least an acceptable or satisfactory version.

In the classroom the teacher can act as a model himself by displaying the attitudes he wishes his students to acquire, or he can provide an outside model in the form of a visiting speaker, a film, a case study, or even a well-told story.

ADVANTAGES

- Can be easily incorporated into the teaching of skills and knowledge.
- Subtle but powerful as long as the model is respected by the students.
- Natural as long as the model displays the attitude honestly.

LIMITATIONS

- If students do not respect or identify with the model, then their attitudes will not be changed positively.
- No one model can be a model for everything.
- The model usually must actually possess the attitude in question. "Faking it" rarely works.

EXAMPLE 1

Two teacher-therapists wanted mental patients to express their feelings more openly and more often during group therapy sessions. Hence, they introduced into the group two patients who displayed the desired behavior. Eventually, other members of the group showed this behavior, apparently as a result of observing the models.

EXAMPLE 2

If a professor of social medicine is enthusiastic, respected, and successful in his work, and if he shows by his actions that he regards social medicine as a crucial issue, it is likely that this attitude will "rub off" on his students. However, it should be noted that an equally esteemed professor of physiology, if he shows little regard for social medicine, can retard the acquisition of this attitude in the same group of medical students.

REFERENCES

Bandura, A.: *Principles of Behavior Modification.* New York: Holt, 1969.

Chapter three contains an extensive discussion of modeling. The author points out that modeling can be a powerful social tool, depending partly on the perceived consequences of the model's behavior.

Luchins, A. S. and Luchins, E. H.: Imitation by rote and understanding. *Journal of Social Psychology. 54:* 175-197, 1961.

This study shows how quickly college students develop a certain behavior after it has been demonstrated by a model and rewarded and how poorly it is acquired when they are merely informed of their errors.

Schwartz, A. N. and Hawkins, H. L.: Patient models and affective statements in group therapy. *Proceedings of the 73rd Annual Convention of the APA.* Washington, D.C.: American Psychological Association, 1965.

In this study the technique of modeling was used in conjunction with rewards, a technique that is described in the next section of this book.

REINFORCING BEHAVIOR

INTRODUCTION One of the dominant themes in social science today is that any given behavior is more likely to reappear when it results in favorable consequences. This viewpoint is not a new one, but in recent years scientists have gained greater understanding of the principles involved.

DESCRIPTION In the following discussion, the term **behavior** refers to observable, measurable actions. Thoughts, feelings, attitudes, and other nonobservable states are not behaviors because they can only be **inferred** from observable behavior. For example, we might infer (although we do not know for certain) that a physician has little respect for a patient if he talks down to that patient, avoids looking directly at him, interrupts him, and disregards his questions.

Modern learning psychologists emphasize that behaviors are strengthened when they are followed by favorable consequences. These consequences are known as rewards or, more technically, as **reinforcement**. A reinforcement is any event, such as praise, a smile, feedback on behavior, or something more tangible, such as money, that increases the likelihood of any given behavior being repeated.

To use the method of **reinforcing behavior** to develop attitudes, a teacher should try to provide some form of reinforcement after the occurrence of student behaviors from which the desired attitudes can be inferred. For example, if an instructor wants students to have a positive attitude toward participating in class discussions, he/she might nod, smile, or say something like "that's a good point" whenever a student does speak up.

PRINCIPLES OF REINFORCING BEHAVIOR

1. *Immediate Reinforcement.* It is important that the reinforcement occur immediately after the desired behavior has been displayed. To use this method effectively, the teacher must provide "on the spot" reactions to student responses, minimizing as much as possible the time between the student's performance and constructive evaluation of that performance.

2. *Shaping Behavior Through Successive Approximations.* Some behaviors must be developed gradually. Rather than expect a sudden change, the instructor may at first need to reinforce each occurrence of a crude semblance of the final, desired behavior. Once this change appears consistently, then reinforcement can be withheld until a still closer approximation of the desired behavior occurs. After a while the more refined behavior will be demonstrated regularly. This process may then be repeated until there is a still more refined form of the desired behavior. In short, according to the principle of shaping, the desired behavior is established gradually, by a series of successive approximations, slowly raising the criterion for reinforcement.

3. *Schedules of reinforcement.* In the early stages, while the behavior is being established by successive approximations, it will develop most rapidly if it is reinforced on each occasion that it appears. Later, when the aim is merely to maintain the already established desirable behavior, reinforcement need not appear on each occasion. In other words, frequent or 100% reinforcement is desirable at first to shape the development of the new behavior, but once it appears regularly, reinforcement can become less frequent. Eventually, "natural" reinforcers (i.e., knowing one is performing correctly) take hold and become effective in sustaining the new behavior, without further intervention by the instructor.

4. *Punishment.* Contrary to what one might expect, undesirable behaviors are **not** always weakened by **un**favorable consequences such as a frown, verbal reprimand, or other form of punishment. The long range effects of punishment are unpredictable; and in the short range, using punishment in an instructional situation with adults is likely to create adverse reactions which will hinder learning.

ADVANTAGES

- Applied correctly, this is one of the most powerful methods of changing attitudes.

- To many instructors, it is "natural" to show approval of desired performance (i.e., to smile, nod, say "good," etc).

LIMITATIONS

- Providing reinforcement for each student at just the right moment may be difficult, especially in a large class of students.

- Can only be used when students are given frequent opportunities to exhibit the desired attitudes.

- Shaping attitudes by providing reinforcement may be a slow process. The instructor must recognize that behavior change may be almost indiscernible at first and that often change in behavior will appear only gradually.

EXAMPLE 1

An instructor in optometry wants his students to adopt the attitude that partially sighted persons must be made to feel at ease in the clinic in order to facilitate successful work with them. The student who, on displaying this attitude, is regularly and immediately reinforced in the form of compliments, high grades, or other recognition continues to develop this attitude. The student who is only occasionally or never rewarded for this attitude may or may not continue to display it.

EXAMPLE 2

An instructor in medical technology wants his students to develop the attitude that the microscope is a high-precision instrument and must be treated with utmost care. Thus, at first, he immediately reinforces his students on every occasion that they are clean and orderly in their work with the microscope. Later, a higher level of performance is encouraged. The student is expected not only to clean the instrument but also to make special adjustments on it with care and finesse, and he is immediately rewarded only when he demonstrates this behavior. Still later, even higher standards are set. Rewards are given only for demonstrating personal initiative in the use and maintenance of his instrutment. Eventually, the student may be expected to encourage others to adopt this general attitude of appreciation in dealing with the microscope, and he is reinforced only when he does so. In this way, complex behavior is built gradually, step by step.

REFERENCES Bandura, A.: *Principles of Behavior Modification*. New York: Holt, 1969.

Chapter four is devoted to the issue of using reinforcement to change behavior. Three sets of variables are seen to be important: (1) developing an incentive system to maintain a high rate of response, (2) making reinforcement conditional on the occurrence of the desired behavior, and (3) using shaping or some similar method to elicit the desired modes of response.

Skinner, B. F.: *Science and Human Behavior*. New York: Macmillan, 1953.

This book is the basic early effort by the leader in this field to demonstrate the role of reinforcement in influencing behavior. All varieties of behavior are considered, ranging from motor skills to verbal behavior to personality development.

GROUP DISCUSSION

DESCRIPTION

In this approach, classes are less formal and the students do more talking than the instructor. Students are allowed to state their views freely. If a class is large, it may be divided into smaller groups to allow more students to exchange more ideas. Group discussion can be used to examine issues, present alternative points of view, and develop communication skills.

ADVANTAGES

- The student's own words, and those of his peers, generally are more influential in changing his attitudes than are the words of the teacher, for two reasons: (1) The student is most likely to notice, remember, and be persuaded by what his friends say, since their approval is often more valued than the approval of the instructor. (2) The student who engages in discussion is actively participating in class, not just listening to the teacher. This active role in class is more conducive to acquiring new, meaningful attitudes than is the passive one of sitting and listening to someone else.

- Group discussion gives the instructor an informal way of assessing existing student attitudes and knowledge.

LIMITATIONS

- Group discussion can be time-consuming, requiring several sessions before any noticeable effect occurs.

- Some students may dominate the discussion while others remain in the background, no more involved than in the lecture approach.

- Popular members of the group may have undesirable attitudes and attempt to persuade others to adopt them.

Note: The solution to these latter two problems lies in the teacher's management of the discussion process. Often, he must guide, direct, or moderate it, but in such a way that the discussion still belongs to the students.

EXAMPLE 1

During the food shortage of the Second World War, the United States government was concerned about the nutrition of the populace. Efforts were made to induce housewives to purchase and serve less-preferred meats of high nutritional value, such as sweetbreads. Two methods were used. One group of housewives listened to a lecture and asked questions of the lecturer, who was a specialist on this topic. Members of the second group spent most of their time in group discussion, where the women talked with one another about the problem. Follow-up studies on two occasions showed that the women who participated in the group discussions later purchased and used the nutritional but less-preferred food more often than did the others.

EXAMPLE 2
Suppose a young health worker attempts to introduce birth-control procedures into a community that practices no family planning. Rather than lecturing on the topic, he might attempt to have a discussion with just a few town leaders, preferably those who are favorable or open-minded about the issue. After these discussions have succeeded, then these "town fathers" might have separate small-group discussions with other members of the town, each time permitting the new people to express their feelings about the proposed changes in their own behavior. In this way, the new ideas are more likely to be accepted.

REFERENCES
Rodin, A. E. and Levine, H. G.: A nonlecture-oriented system of pathology education: Rationale, experiences and analysis. *Journal of Medical Education. 48:* 349-355, 1973.

Medical students obtained the basic information in this pathology course via a textbook while the faculty provided opportunities for group discussions, enrichment and problem-solving. The results showed that the students not only gained greater knowledge of pathology but also gained a significantly more positive attitude toward the relevancy of studying pathology.

ROLE PLAYING

DESCRIPTION

An individual's role is his function in a group, such as secretary of a committee, member of a class, or coach of a team. In role playing, a person temporarily adopts a specified role and tries to behave in ways characteristic of a person in that role.

In the health fields, role playing usually involves having one student take the part of a specific health worker, for instance, a nutritionist working with low-income patients, and having another student play the role of a patient in that context. Both are given a setting or situation in which to interact.

ADVANTAGES

- Role playing offers students a chance to try out real-world attitudes and behaviors, ones that otherwise might be inappropriate or unavailable to him.

- Role playing is usually thought to be fun for the students.

- Playing roles opposite to one's usual role (e.g., patient instead of professional) helps students develop empathy with that opposing role which can be important to professional performance.

LIMITATIONS

- Role playing depends heavily on the student's imagination and capacity to project himself into another situation.

- Role playing can be time-consuming, especially if repeated many times with students playing a variety of roles.

EXAMPLE 1

In one instance researchers created an opportunity for teachers to engage in role playing in the hope that they would thereby develop a more positive attitude toward using role playing in their own teaching. The setting was the faculty lounge and the issue at hand, established only for purposes of role playing, was a proposed new curriculum. One teacher was assigned the role of presenting the new curriculum; another was designated as the typically hostile colleague; two more were assigned to be close friends of one another; another was designated as "group worrier"; another was the inevitable "discussion blocker"; and still others, reluctant to engage in role playing themselves at this first exposure, were assigned as observers, to record and report what occurred during the learning session.

The hostile colleague played his role excellently and all participants seemed thoroughly involved. Afterward, as indicated in a follow-up evaluation, it appeared that the participants had a much more favorable attitude toward using this technique themselves in their own classrooms.

EXAMPLE 2

A student nurse may learn to have more confidence in her future capacity as a health team member if she is allowed to play the role of team nurse while others in the class act as the social worker, physician, family member, and hospital administrator.

EXAMPLE 3 Similarly, a medical student, in dealing with a classmate may observe an abruptness in that classmate's manner. After such an experience, he will probably try to avoid that type of abruptness in his own behavior with patients in the future.

REFERENCES Chesler, M. and Fox, R.: *Role Playing Methods in the Classroom.* Chicago: SRA, 1966.

This booklet, from the Center for Research on the Utilization of Scientific Knowledge at the University of Michigan, describes the theoretical foundations of role playing, case studies, the basic techniques, and methods of evaluating role playing outcomes.

Janis, I. L.: Attitude change via role playing. In R. P. Abelson et al. (Eds.): *Theories of Cognitive Consistency: A Sourcebook.* Chicago: Rand McNally, 1968.

A rather technical discussion in the context of social psychological theory, especially cognitive dissonance.

Moreno, J. L.: *Psychodrama.* New York: Beacon House, 1946.

This book, by a rather flambouyant writer, is responsible for initiating much of the modern interest in role playing in education and therapy. The therapeutic method called psychodrama is based on role playing.

SIMULATION GAMES

DESCRIPTION

Classroom games usually involve a simulation of real-world situations and processes, often in a simplified but dramatic manner. Unlike formal games, such as chess and monopoly, in games designed for educational purposes the **process** of play is more important than the **outcome**.

The following formats have been used in simulation games:

1. *Problem-solving exercises.* Games that provide a framework for solving a particular type of problem, generally by posing a specific problem and specifying a sequence of steps for solving that problem. For example, formulating a goal, assigning priorities, allocating resources, and then distributing them.

2. *Board games.* In these games, ideas or processes are represented by means of concrete symbols: chips, markers, and a game board. Students investigate the processes by manipulating the symbols.

3. *Computer-assisted games.* Here the computer is used to perform any of three functions to aid players: calculations, storage and retrieval of information, and feedback of a mathematical or nonmathematical nature about players' judgments and decisions.

Simulation games involve elements of two previously described methods, group discussion and role playing. An important difference among the three lies in the degree of structure. Usually there is the least structure in group discussion; there are some implicit behavior patterns to be followed in role playing; and in simulation games there are usually explicit rules to be obeyed, which are similar to the regulations and procedures in an actual setting outside the classroom.

ADVANTAGES

- Can strengthen human interaction skills as well as process skills such as planning, decision making, and thinking "on your feet," all of which have a strong attitudinal component.

- When games are done well, students become highly motivated and involved.

- Students receive immediate feedback on the consequences of their decisions.

- Once the rules of a game are well established, students often can proceed without further assistance from the instructor.

LIMITATIONS

- Game play may involve considerable instructional time.

- Preparation of the game (i.e., establishing the rules of play and developing the necessary supportive materials) usually requires considerable effort on the part of the instructor.

EXAMPLE 1 (A PROBLEM- SOLVING EXERCISE)	In a game called EDPLAN, students are divided into three or more teams or groups, each competing against the others. The game is focused around the educational issues of school planning and financial problems. Each team plays the game by deciding on its priorities in these areas and then allocating portions of the fixed budget to these priorities. The program and budget of each team is studied and rated by the others. Determining a winner is not important. The learning and attitude change emerge more from the process of playing the game than from the final outcome.
EXAMPLE 2 (A BOARD GAME)	Another game, called Planafam, illustrates the relationship between social conditions and the family planning behavior of individuals. It emphasizes the need for fertility control and the ways in which it can be achieved. The only playing materials are a board and cards. One to 12 people can play simultaneously, and players can be formed into teams to accommodate still larger numbers. Successful play is based on strategic thinking, decision making, compromising, and role playing, although chance is intentionally included as a significant factor.
EXAMPLE 3 (A PROBLEM- SOLVING EXERCISE)	A game for students if hospital administration requires that students divide themselves into groups of specialists, such as nurses, surgeons, maintenance personnel, social workers, and so forth. The classroom represents a full meeting of the hospital council where each group of specialists vies for a larger section of the budget and more physical space in the building. If all the students playing this game are able to work out their viewpoints thoroughly, perhaps as a homework assignment, the simulated council session can become quite lively and students will observe the potential for rivalries, grievances, and perceived injustices in a hospital setting. The speeches, rebuttals, and discussions of their classmates should help them acquire a more realistic attitude about the future problems they will face as hospital administrators.

REFERENCES

Abt, C.: *Serious Games.* New York: Viking Press, 1970.

This book describes the use of games specifically for instructional purposes. Many types and levels are illustrated, from elementary school to professional level; guidelines for the development of games are included.

Gordon, A. K.: *Games for Growth.* Chicago: SRA, 1970.

A readable, broad introduction to the use of games in the classroom. Chapter seven focuses on teaching attitudes through games.

Twelker, P. A. (Ed.): *Instructional Simulation Systems: An Annotated Bibliography.* Corvallis, Ore.: Continuing Education Publications, 1969.

This source is a bibliography by a well-known writer in this field.

Zuckerman, D. W. and Horn, R. E.: *The Guide to Simulations/Games for Education and Training.* P.O. Box 417, Lexington, Mass., Information Resources Inc., 1973.

This continually updated guide includes a chapter on Simulations for the Health Professions. Several general articles on simulation/games are included as well. An excellent source of games that have already been developed and are available for purchase.

REAL-WORLD EXPERIENCES

DESCRIPTION

Sometimes it is possible for the instructor to help his students develop certain attitudes by arranging for them to experience specific aspects of the world outside the classroom. Usually these experiences involve exposure to conditions normally experienced by patients of the health professionals being trained.

EXAMPLE 1

One method of helping medical students develop greater sensitivity to the experience of the patient in an ambulatory setting is to assign them to visit a clinic and wait among the patients for several hours.

EXAMPLE 2

Nutrition students have been required to use a diet that later they would prescribe for others. This experience helps them to develop a more realistic attitude about the problems a patient encounters in following a diet prescribed by a nutritionist or physician.

EXAMPLE 3

A group of mental health practitioners once committed themselves to a mental hospital. Their purpose was to increase their awareness of conditions in that institution.

ADVANTAGES

- The attitudes acquired in this context are likely to be stronger, more realistic, and more meaningful than most of those acquired in a classroom setting.

LIMITATIONS

- Arranging the real-world experiences may require a great deal of time and effort.

- Effective use of real-world experiences usually depends on careful preparation, structuring, and follow-up by the instructor.

REFERENCES

Bennett, J. F., Saxton, G. A., Lutwama, J. S. W., and Namboze, M. B.: The role of a rural health center in the teaching program of a medical school in East Africa. *Journal of Medical Education. 40*: 690-699, 1965.

By working and learning in a rural health center, medical students developed attitudes that the authors felt would be beneficial in work situations in East Africa.

Holzberg, J. D. and Knapp, R. H.: The social interaction of college students and chronically ill mental patients. *American Journal of Orthopsychiatry. 35*: 473-492, 1965.

This article describes a year-long experiment in exposing college students to diverse social contacts with mental patients.

Miles, J. E., Maurice, W. L., and Krell, R.: The student psychiatric ward: An innovative teaching approach for medical undergraduates. *Journal of Medical Education. 49*: 176-181, 1974.

In this study fourth-year medical students were the only medical staff in two psychiatric units. No adverse patient response was observed while the students reported significant gains in their capacity to appreciate the patient's circumstances.

Wallace, S.: *Curriculum Design Project in Nutrition.* Boston: Harvard School of Public Health, Teacher Preparation Program, Unpublished, 1974.

METHODS FOR GROUP INSTRUCTION

INTRODUCTION   The instructional methods described in this section are useful when teaching groups of students in classroom situations. This is true also of the methods for developing attitudes which are discussed in the previous section. However, whereas the primary instructional function of the methods in the previous section is "shaping student attitudes," the methods described here have primarily other instructional functions, as will be indicated for each method.

DIRECTORY

LECTURE

DESCRIPTION

An instructional method of presentation using the speaker as the primary mode of transmission. May be supported by audiovisual media.

INSTRUCTIONAL FUNCTIONS SERVED

- Providing a frame of reference (i.e., introductions, overviews, etc).
- Transmitting information.
- Providing a reason to learn (but only if instructor is a dynamic speaker).

ADVANTAGES

- Can present substantial amounts of information to large numbers of people in short periods of time, with minimum cost and delay.
- Can present up-to-date information not otherwise available—descriptions of work in progress, recent research, for example.

LIMITATIONS

- Capable of providing only a low level of simulation.
- Frequently the information recorded in student notes is incomplete and inaccurate: However, lectures can be audio- or video-taped for student review and/or repeat presentations.
- Demonstrations accompanying lectures are frequently difficult to see in large audience situations.
- Extensive student participation is not possible.
- Difficult to make provision for differences in student background or learning style.

REFERENCES

Bughman, E.: The lecture method of instruction. *Development of Educational Programmes for the Health Professions.* Geneva, World Health Organization, 1973.

A systems approach to planning the lecture is advocated. Consideration must be given to entry-level knowledge and the formulation of behavioral judged objectives. Two-way communication is essential. Skills in opening and closing a lecture are cited, and the use of visual aids is discussed. It is submitted that lectures are useful in helping students to acquire information, but less efficient in promoting problem-solving skills or attitudinal goals than the seminars, discussions, tutorials, or other student-centered activities.

Miller, G. E. (Ed.): *Teaching and Learning in Medical School,* Cambridge, Mass., Harvard University Press, 1968.

Contains a section on the use of the lecture in medical education, its advantages and disadvantages.

McCabe, B. P. and Bender, C. C.: *Speaking is a Practical Matter*. Boston, Holbrook Press, 1968.

A readable text designed to increase one's competency as a speaker.

Center for Disease Control: *Lecture Preparation Guide.* U.S. Government Printing Office, Public Health Service Publication, No. 1421, 1969.

Concise procedural guidelines for planning and implementing a lecture.

McCleish, J.: *The Lecture Method.* Cambridge, England: Institute of Education, 1968.

Opinion research in which teachers stated that on the whole lecturing was a valuable mode of instruction, while students felt that lectures were overrated and ineffective as a means of communicating knowledge. Less than 40% recall was shown immediately after university lectures, recall was less for delayed tests.

PROGRAMMED LECTURE

INTRODUCTION   The programmed lecture is an instructional technique that bridges the gap between the traditional lecture in which information is transmitted primarily by a speaker and programmed instruction in which the learner systematically interacts with instructional materials that are logically constructed toward specific measurable objectives. The programmed lecture is organized primarily for retrieval of information by the learner.

DESCRIPTION   An instructional method using learner feedback as a device for monitoring student learning. The instructor planning and implementing a programmed lecture:

1. Establishes objectives for the lecture.

2. Attempts to justify all selected content by asking, "If I want to present this particular information, what change in behavior do I want to produce? Specifically, how can I test for this behavior?" Test items are prepared for each important point.

3. Insures quick response by the learner and immediate feedback by constructing test items that

   - are relevant to the information to be learned,

   - are restricted in number, usually no more than 10 per 50-minute lecture,

   - are brief,

   - avoid ambiguity,

   - require short answers or multiple-choice responses.

4. Presents test items in a format visible to all learners simultaneously. Projected 35 mm slides or overhead transparencies are commonly used, but large lettered placards may be used if projection is not feasible.

5. Intersperses test items at logical but irregular intervals to keep learners attentive.

6. Provides immediate reinforcement to student responses by commenting on right and wrong responses.

   Learner response to the lecturer may be provided by:

   - A show of hands for each of several alternative answers.

   - An electronic response system which provides immediate individual and group data.

- Large (10 x 10) cards with a different color on each margin are displayed to the lecturer by all students simultaneously according to their test item choices. Instructor can tell immediately how many students answered the question correctly.

- Providing test items on individual sheets with space for notes by the learner. This system provides delayed feedback to the lecturer when he analyzes student responses.

INSTRUCTIONAL
FUNCTIONS
SERVED

- Transmitting information.

- Providing feedback on student progress.

- Allowing students to practice.

ADVANTAGES

- Active responding and feedback promotes learner attention.

- Electronic response systems permit maximum learner response, privacy, immediate feedback to both lecturer and learner, and individual response data to the lecturer for detailed analysis.

- Paper-and-pencil response format allows short answer as well as multiple-choice test item formats. It may also provide a good course review mechanism.

DISADVANTAGES

- Course preparation is relatively arduous and time-consuming.

- Electronic response systems are expensive to purchase and maintain.

- Electronic and coded card response systems restrict test-item format to multiple choice.

- Individual learner color-coded response cards permit only partial learner privacy, and feedback to the instructor, although immediate, provides group response only.

- Paper-and-pencil response system provides delayed feedback to the lecturer.

- Generally limits amount of material that can be presented.

REFERENCES

Barnhard, H. J.: A typical programmed instruction: two case reports. *J. Med. Ed. 46*: 464-465, 1971.

Presents three different formats for different types of groups in a medical education setting (radiology). The learner responds with paper and pencil. Anonymous papers are collected and graded by the lecturer. Provides feedback to both the learner and the lecturer.

Bridgman, C. F., Matzke, H. A.: Innovations in the teaching of anatomy. *Am. J. Vet. Res. 26*: 1552-1561, 1965.

Focuses on use of an electronic responder for lecture presentation. Suggests incorporating a responder in the multi-media setting of the anatomy laboratory for more effective learning.

Deterline, W. A.: Practical problems in program production. *Programmed Instruction.* P. C. Lange (Ed.): National Society for the Study of Education, Chicago, University of Chicago Press. Chap. VII, 1967.

This chapter deals with likely bases for advancement of programmed instruction. It includes a section entitled "Programming for the class-room" or "Programmed lesson plans." A broader view of the principles and variations of the programmed lecture than described in the other references cited here.

Ludwig, J.: Medical school teachers—there is a message from an airline. *J. Dent. Ed. 37:* 13-15, 1973.

A programmed lecture system based on simple color-card response. Sets forth common system for eliminating distracting concurrent note-taking.

McCarthy, W. H.: Improving large audience teaching: the programmed lecture. *Brit. J. Med. Ed. 4:* 29-31, 1970.

A programmed lecture system utilizing an answer sheet response system with no teacher feedback. Provides useful review format for students. Questions are structured according to programming principles. Surgery application.

GUEST INTERVIEW

INTRODUCTION The guest interview is an alternative to the traditional use of guest lecturers, which is often unsuccessful for one or more of the following reasons:

- The lecturer may cover points that have already been covered in the course or omit points you wanted him/her to cover.

- The standard lecture method makes it difficult to dovetail the contributions of several visiting speakers.

- Once started, a lecturer is likely to "follow his own trajectory" regardless of the original agreement.

- Some invited experts may turn out to be poor lecturers.

DESCRIPTION A **guest interview** involves having the instructor or course participants direct a series of prearranged questions to the invited speaker. The interview conforms to the natural flow of conversation rather than to any formal questioning procedure.

Arranging for the Interview

1. The instructor selects the areas in the curriculum where it seems desirable to involve outside speakers and chooses possible speakers.

2. The instructor then contacts the speakers, tells them of the interest in interviewing them, describes the interview method, and requests each guest's relevant publications.

3. The instructor reviews the speaker's publications and draws up a tentative list of questions to be asked in the interview (this may be done in collaboration with students).

4. The list is submitted to the guest speaker, who is asked to make modifications, deletions, and additions. This process can be accomplished on the phone or by letter and serves to reassure the guest as well as communicate the specific requirements for the session. It also permits the guest speaker to anticipate sensitive questions. The final, agreed on list of questions forms the basis for the interview.

Conducting the Interview

1. The instructor: Reviews the agreement with the speaker beforehand so the speaker won't be annoyed or surprised by the technique.

2. Allows the speaker to warm up to his subject: starts with 3 or 4 minutes of self-introduction by the speaker and a few specific questions dealing with the context of the interview.

3. Does not allow the interview to continue for the entire instruction period; allows time for class participation and exchange with the guest.

4. Steers the speaker away from stereotyped statements. Probing statements such as: "well, I am not quite certain that I know what you mean by that. Would you explain a little further" may be effective here.

5. Keeps the visitor giving short, sharp replies.

6. Allows the dialogue to develop naturally.

7. Keeps the guest on the subject.

INSTRUCTIONAL FUNCTIONS SERVED	• Transmitting information. • Providing a reason to learn (if guest is dynamic).
ADVANTAGES	• Guests like the method because they do not have to prepare a lecture. • Assures continuity within the course. • Allows instructor to maintain control over the presentation. • Allows instructor to draw on experts in area being discussed. • Provides for student participation.
DISADVANTAGES	• Some people cannot adjust to the give and take of an interview. • Certain content areas, a careful sequential account for example, do not lend themselves to this approach.
EXAMPLE	The following questions were used in a guest interview by Dr. Gerald Caplan, Harvard Medical School.

1. Please describe briefly the City Hospital Center at Elmhurst at the time you set up the Trouble-Shooting Clinic. What size population did it serve? Did it have an official or unofficial "catchment area?" Briefly describe the nature of the population, ethnically, socially, culturally, etc. What mental health facilities were available to them and how did they utilize these?

2. What were your goals in setting up the Trouble-Shooting Clinic?

3. Please give a brief description of the life-history of the project? How did you set up the Trouble-Shooting Clinic? What relation did it have to the rest of your program and to the other services of the hospital? How was it received by your own staff and your hospital and community colleagues? What factors led to its closure?

4. Describe in detail the way the Trouble-Shooting Clinic operated.

5. What were the community contacts of the Trouble-Shooting Clinic?

6. Discuss the flow of cases through the Trouble-Shooting Clinic during its existence from 1958 to 1964. Were there any significant changes in the number and types of cases? Were these changes related to changes in the policies and practices of you and your staff?

7. How did you keep abreast of the flow of cases, or did you develop waiting lists for treatment or dispositional decision? Describe your techniques of rapid diagnosis and brief psychotherapy.

8. Describe and discuss your studies to demonstrate the degree of achievement of your goals, with particular reference to secondary prevention, i.e., reduction in prevalence by reduction in duration of a significant proportion of the mentally disordered in your population.

CASE METHOD

DESCRIPTION

The *case method* utilizes a factual history or description of an event written from the vantage point and using the facts available to one observer.

Case studies are structured and used in several different ways in teaching. Before reading a case it is important to determine how it is supposed to be used in class and for what purpose.

1. *Case Histories as Examples:* Cases may be used as examples to support a point the instructor is trying to make. The lecturer points out general principles that held true in the case under study. The student is a more or less a passive listener. Class time is largely taken up by the instructor telling what the case "means."

2. *Class-Dominated Case Studies:* Students play an active role; the instructor moderates discussion. Several methods may be used:

   - *Cliff hanger cases:* Students are asked to read a case that outlines a complex situation and includes a problem calling for a decision. The case narrative stops at the decision point, and students are asked what they would do and why. In class, students defend the factual basis and reasoning that led to their decision.

   - *Incident type cases:* Students are presented with short descriptions (i.e., 100-200 words) of a problem situation. If they ask the right questions, they are supplied with more information. As a group, students take the role of the decision-maker trying to straighten out the problem. Sometimes they are divided into teams (example: union team versus management team) and asked to defend their respective positions; however, the class must come to a decision that is mutually agreeable. In many ways incident-type cases are similar to simulations.

   - *Case histories to stimulate inductive or deductive reasoning:* Some instructors ask students to read and analyze a case, by answering a series of questions about the case. Cases used in these situations are usually **not** "cliff hangers." Less emphasis is placed on what action should be taken to solve an immediate problem, and more on understanding the development of the problem and its solution.

INSTRUCTIONAL FUNCTIONS SERVED

- Allowing students to practice problem-solving and decision-making skills.
- Providing feedback.
- Providing a reason to learn.

ADVANTAGES
- Students tend to like this method, since realistic cases are intrinsically interesting.
- Students learn from classmates as well as from the instructor.
- Gives students practice in thinking of themselves in the roles they will later fill.
- Active participation and back-and-forth dialogues keep classes interesting.

DISADVANTAGES
- Students who are not used to this method may initially experience frustration with the lack of direction and feel they are wasting their time. (Proponents of the case method claim that this period is followed by an arousal of curiosity, development of insight, and finally by the development of a great deal more administrative skill than with lecture-type teaching.)
- Some subjects (e.g., biochemistry) cannot be easily taught by a series of cases.
- Progress in development of problem-solving and administrative skills is slow.
- Usually a case study assumes a basic knowledge of the facts and certain skills as well as maturity and readiness to accept responsibility.
- Case studies may over-emphasize positive decisions when sometimes negative decisions or holding-waiting actions are the best policy.
- Cases tend to oversimplify real-world situations, because including all the variables actually involved would make them too long or cumbersome.

SOURCES OF CASES

American Board of Orthopedic Surgery, in conjunction with The Center for the Study of Medical Education, University of Illinois College of Medicine, Chicago, Illinois

Publishes cases in patient management.

Intercollegiate Case Clearing House
Soldiers Field Road
Boston, Mass. 02163

Publishes cases in health policy and health services administration.

REFERENCES

Intercollegiate Case Clearing House: *Abstracts of Cases for Teaching Health Services Administration.* Boston: Intercollegiate Case Clearing House, 1972.

An annotated listing of case method materials available for teachers of health services administration.

McNair, M. P. and Hersum, A. C. (Eds.): *The Case Method at the Harvard Business School.* New York: McGraw-Hill, 1954.

A collection of papers on the philosophy, use, and writing of cases for business education.

Penchansky, R.: *Health Services Administration: Policy Cases and the Case Method.* Cambridge, Mass.: Harvard University Press, 1968.

A collection of 12 case studies for use in training health services administrators. Cases focus on policy issues, planning, and evaluation, using topics such as nationalized health services, union medical care programs, and community health services administration.

Sprague, L., Sheldon, A., and McLaughlin, C.: *Teaching Health and Human Services Administration by the Case Method.*
New York: Behavioral Publications, 1973.

Describes uses that cases can have in health services curricula, the classroom dynamics pertaining to their use, and the development of case materials. Extensive annotated listing of case materials already available in health administration is included.

Pigors, P. and Pigors, F.: *Case Method in Human Relations: The Incident Process.* New York: McGraw-Hill, 1961.

Use of the case method to analyze social situations. Examples of cases from personnel administration and academic settings.

Pigors, P., Pigors, R., and Tribou, M.: *Professional Nursing Practice, Cases and Issues.* New York: McGraw-Hill, 1967.

Ten cases for nursing education, concerning social interaction and decision-making.

TRIGGER FILMS

Trigger films are short vignette films that are designed to stimulate audience reaction. Their purpose is to elicit an emotional response in the viewer(s) and "trigger" meaningful group discussion of the issues portrayed.

They encourage the viewer to supply his own interpretation and have been likened to Rorschach tests on film. They are often used in opening discussion on topics that students may be initially reluctant to probe.

Trigger films are brief and to the point. They present only part of an event and end before the resolution of the problem is reached. The viewer is left to reconstruct the beginning and predict the outcome.

Situations portrayed in trigger films represent issues that are emotionally charged for most people, yet the films themselves do not attempt to put forth value judgments. Since they leave much unsaid, the viewer is encouraged to project his own feelings and expectations into the situation.

Most trigger films portray, realistically, everyday experiences with which the audience can identify. People may tend to react defensively when they see "themselves" portrayed in a negative light. Caricaturing or exaggerating the characters so that a comfortable distance is established between the protagonists and the viewer may prevent negative audience response.

Trigger films are most effective when discussion follows immediately after showing the film. The group leader does not force the discussion, but allows the group to formulate opinions and solutions. The viewers are informed ahead of time that there are no "correct" solutions.

INSTRUCTIONAL FUNCTIONS SERVED
- Providing a reason to learn.
- Shaping student attitudes.

ADVANTAGES
- Can be used to stimulate thinking on **interpersonal behavior** of which the health professional must be conscious in his own practice. Examples of positive or negative relationships with patients or colleagues can be portrayed to stimulate awareness among students.

- Can function as **problem-oriented teaching materials**, providing unresolved case examples to which students must apply their own creativity and knowledge to "solve."

- Portions of longer films can be used.

- Provides a common focus for student discussion.

- May be replayed if audience disagrees on what happened.

LIMITATIONS

- Trigger films are **not** intended to transmit information by themselves—the real learning takes place in the ensuing discussion. They are not designed to demonstrate appropriate procedures or models but, instead to stimulate discussion through which these concepts can come to light.

- Leading and directing the ensuing discussion may be difficult to structure and manage for teachers not skilled in leading discussions.

EXAMPLE

The Center for Educational Development at the University of Illinois College of Medicine has produced a series of trigger films for use in orthopedic residency programs. One of these depicts an incident during ward rounds at which a patient's condition is discussed in a callous way by the attending physician, in the patient's presence. The patient is silent throughout, ignored, while the attending physician calls on his students to diagnose the case.

Other trigger films have been produced on drug use by teenagers, driving safety, problems of the aging, dentistry, mental retardation, and teacher education.

SOURCES OF TRIGGER FILMS

American Dental Association. Bureau of Dental Health Education, Chicago, Ill.

Films on patient education and preventive dentistry.

Bureau of Health Manpower Education. National Medical Audiovisual Center, Atlanta, Ga.

Films on health manpower needs.

Center for Educational Development. University of Illinois College of Medicine, Chicago, Ill.

Films on patient management produced for orthopedic residency programs.

Dental Manpower Development Center. Louisville, Ke.

Films on the management of auxiliary personnel.

Inter-University Film Group. University of Missouri, Kansas City, Mo.

A series of twenty problem-centered 'stimulus films' for teacher education.

London Hospital Medical College. Dental School, London, England.

Films on oral health care for children.

Television Center. University of Michigan, Ann Arbor, Mich.

Trigger films for use with young drivers, produced for the Highway Safety Research Institute, University of Michigan (1968).

"Project 72" and "Project 119"—films for use with teachers and prospective teachers of dentistry (1969 and 1972).

Films for use at the 1971 White House Conference on Aging.

Trigger films on drugs (1970).

Trigger films on Mental Retardation and the Law, for the University of Michigan Institute for the Study of Mental Retardation.

REFERENCES

Fisch, A. L.: The trigger film technique. *Improving College and University Teaching.* 286-289, Fall 1970.

Discusses the concept of trigger films and their use in the teaching of attitudes. Suggestions for production and use of trigger films. Bibliography lists agencies which have produced films on various health topics.

Gliessman, D. and Williams, D. G.: Stimulus films—films made from pretested scripts as a medium for teacher education. *Audiovisual Instruction. 11*: 552-554, September 1966.

The use of trigger films as problem-centered instructional materials in educational psychology. Those film topics which would be most useful were determined by a survey of the opinions of students, education instructors, and practicing teachers.

Gliessman, D. and Williams, D. G.: *Inter-University Film Project: The Production of Five Stimulus Films to Be Used in Teacher Education. Final Report.* University of Missouri at Kansas City. (ERIC Microfiche # ED 015-644.) January 1967.

Report on the development of five problem-centered films for teacher education. The themes of the films, which dramatize realistic teaching problems, are stated along with a series of questions and exercises for use with each film.

Miller, E. J.: Trigger filmmaking. *Audiovisual Instruction, 16*: 64-67, May 1971.

Production of trigger films at the University of Michigan Television Center on drug use, aging, and legal problems of the mentally retarded. Brief suggestions for producing such films.

Olson, C. J.: The use of 'trigger films' in discussion groups. *AHME Journal*, 9-13, November-December 1971.

Discusses films produced by the Center for Educational Development at the University of Illinois College of Medicine, and lists suggestions for preparing trigger films. One example described.

METHODS FOR INDIVIDUALIZED INSTRUCTION

INTRODUCTION   This section describes a variety of methods for adapting the instructional process to individual students, or for allowing students more control over what and how they learn than is generally afforded by group-paced methods of instruction.

DIRECTORY

INDIVIDUALIZING INSTRUCTION: OVERVIEW

DESCRIPTION

Instruction is said to be individualized when its contents, sequence, pace and/or methods are modified to conform to variations in the learner's present knowledge, ability, interests, or learning style.

Instruction can be individualized in many ways, most of which remove the teacher from the center of the stage. Emphasis is placed on having each student learn at his own pace in his own way. The instructor becomes a coach, a counselor, a leader of small groups, or a director of individual projects.

BEST INSTRUCTIONAL USE

Experimental evidence has shown that individualized instruction is more effective than group-paced instruction when one or both of the following prevail:

1. *Student heterogeneity*—when students differ widely in backgrounds, interests, abilities, and/or future professional goals.
2. *Independent learning styles*—when students as a group tend to be self-confident, self-initiated, and high-risk-takers (as opposed to being generally dependent on rewards offered within the classroom, low on self-propulsion, etc).

TECHNIQUE FOR MANAGING INDIVIDUALIZED INSTRUCTION

It is generally easier to individualize instruction when the **student-teacher** ratio is low. However, individualization can be accomplished even when a high student-teacher ratio prevails by dividing students into small groups and/or using selected students as **teaching assistants**. (See "Use of Teaching Assistants," Page C-93).

Another technique which is useful for managing individualized instruction is the **grade contract**, whereby each student contracts with the teacher for a specific grade in exchange for specified performance on the part of that student (see "Grade Contracts," page C-94).

The table on the following page summarizes a variety of ways in which instruction can be personalized or adapted to individual learning styles.

TECHNIQUES FOR INDIVIDUALIZING INSTRUCTION

VARIABLE	SUGGESTED METHODS
Content	1. Allow students as a group or individually to select those objectives they want to achieve from a prepared set of possible objectives. 2. Suggest a wide range of topics for individual projects or allow students to select project of own interest. 3. Offer "reading," "tutorial," or "supervised research" components. 4. Provide remedial and/or advanced segments for different student proficiencies. 5. Divide class into small interest groups which then pursue different topics or objectives.
Sequence	1. Allow students as a group to choose the order in which the class will cover a set of objectives. 2. Develop self-instructional packages for each objective or logical grouping of objectives, and allow students to go through the materials in whatever order they choose. (See "Learning Packages," page C-113).
Pace	1. Allow students to set their own deadlines for meeting specific objectives; for example, for turning in various parts of a research proposal. 2. Allow students to take tests and exams whenever they are ready instead of at a scheduled time. 3. Assign units of programmed instruction that students may work through at their own pace. (See "Programmed Instruction: Overview," beginning on page C-97).
Methods	1. Set up several "tracks" or ways in which students can reach the same objectives; for example, reading text plus attending lectures or working through a set of programmed materials and viewing several videotapes. (See "Learning Packages," page C-113). 2. Set up an area in library or audiovisual center that will allow students to examine and use functionally equivalent ways of reaching the same objectives. 3. Allow students as a group or individually to select those instructional activities they wish to pursue to achieve designated instructional objectives.

REFERENCES   Edling, J. V.: *Individualized Instruction: A Manual for Administrators.* Corvallis, Oregon: D.C.E. Publishers, n.d.

A description of various options for individualizing instruction. Examples from elementary and secondary education. Good summary of experimental data regarding the effectiveness of individualized instruction in the classroom.

Gronlund, N. E.: *Individualizing Classroom Instruction.* New York: MacMillan, 1974.

Individualized Instruction Systems are described and classified in terms of the degree of the students' freedom of choice. Excellent summary of the state of the art in this area. Good bibliography.

USE OF TEACHING ASSISTANTS

DESCRIPTION

Teaching assistants are usually advanced students who have taken previous courses in the subject and whose talents can be utilized to individualize and refine instruction. Assistants may take one or more of these roles:

— Lead small group discussion.
— Review work individually with students.
— Guide student efforts in laboratory exercises.
— Evaluate written work of students.
— Assist in the design of course materials.
— Give feedback to the instructor regarding progress of students and regarding the effectiveness of the teaching plan and the course materials.

To use teaching assistants, the instructor should:

(a) select individuals who will profit from the teaching experience and who have indicated an interest in teaching;
(b) prepare the teaching assistants for their roles by providing opportunity for assistants to work through the course materials and interact with the instructor regarding both substantive questions, and questions of course logistics; and
(c) hold regular staff meetings to go over session plans, student problems, or problems with the course materials.

ADVANTAGES

● Provides an inexpensive way of assuring a favorable student/teacher ratio.

● Facilitates individualizing instruction by allowing students to interact in small groups.

● Gives the individual contemplating a teaching career an opportunity to carry out clearly prescribed teaching functions in a relatively unstressful situation.

● Teaching assistants learn both substantive and teaching skills as they work with students.

LIMITATIONS

● Training teaching assistants requires expenditure of time and effort, which must be repeated for each cycle.

● Planning a course utilizing teaching assistants requires careful logistic planning of activities.

● Teachers' guides and session plans must be prepared in advance so that all teaching assistants are working towards the goals and objectives of the course.

GRADE CONTRACTS

DESCRIPTION

A grade contract is a written agreement between the instructor and a student which states that the student will receive a specified grade on completion of specified requirements. By signing such a grade contract **before** the course or unit of instruction, the student agrees to fulfill certain objectives for a particular grade, and the instructor agrees to award this grade if the student attains the performance level specified.

Course requirements might be met by one or several contracts. A grade contract usually includes explanations of:

- the purpose and value of the unit;

- the instructional objectives of the contract and the criteria for determining if the objectives have been met;

- the means by which the student will achieve these objectives;

- the testing situation and the requirements for passing the test;

- pertinent or recommended resources.

During contract negotiation, standards of mastery can usually be adjusted to the needs and abilities of the individual student; but once agreed on, the contract is binding.

Since one of the purposes of grade contracts is to minimize anxiety over grades, the student is usually given as many chances as he needs to work through the contract and satisfy the objectives.

Flexibility is afforded through the use of both teacher-made and student-made contracts. At the beginning of the course the instructor will probably want to design most of the contracts. As students gain familiarity with the course material and with contracting, designing their own contracts affords them the opportunity to explore areas of special interest.

ADVANTAGES

- Particularly useful for self-directed learners who like to be in control of the learning process.

- Minimizes grade anxiety and competitiveness.

- Minimizes subjective and arbitrary grading procedures, assuming, of course, the contract incorporates objective evaluation criteria and procedures for applying them.

- Students can gain experience in self-evaluation and can take some responsibility for their own learning and growth.

LIMITATIONS
- Time is needed to prepare contracts and to coach students in their use.

- Does not provide incentive for self-directed activity peripheral to the contract. Student may not be motivated to do more than the contract requires.

- If the contract is considered to be binding, it does not provide a mechanism for timid students who aim low initially to improve their grade if confidence is gained in mid-course. (Alternatively, contract renegotiation may be permitted and encouraged.)

REFERENCES

Anon.: Behavioral objectives and student learning contracts in the teaching of economics. *Journal of Economic Education. 4*: 43-49, Fall 1972.

Ties in the desirability of specifying students' goals in demonstrable or measurable terms (behavioral objectives with the concept of designing grade contracts written in terms of such objectives. Examples given from the teaching of economics.

Dash, E.: Contract for grades. *The Clearing House. 45*: 231-235, December 1970.

Points out that grade contracts encourage students' sense of responsibility for their own work. A sample contract is presented, and cautions in the use of contracts are given.

Esbensen, T.: The Duluth Contract: What it is and what it does. *Educational Technology. 12*: 22-23, September 1972.

A sample contract is given and its components analyzed.

Harvey, A.: Contracts—A break in the grading game. *Education Canada. 12:* 40-44, September 1972.

A short introduction to the concept of grade contracts, pointing out some of its attractions and drawbacks.

Lewis, L. A., and Devore, E.: Contract grading: An alliance for learning. *Journal of Dental Education. 35:* 24-28, October 1971.

The concept of grade contracts is discussed in relation to the types of objectives desired; components of a contract and suggestions for their design are presented; advantages of grade contracts for the student, the instructor, and for the professional curriculum.

Lloyd, K. E., and Knutzen, N. J.: A self-paced programmed undergraduate course in the experimental analysis of behavior. *Journal of Applied Behavior Analysis. 2*: 125-133, Summer 1969.

Describes a course in which grades were earned through an explicit, nonarbitrary point-accumulation system, but without the device of grade contracts. (An example of an alternative grading system.)

Stewart, J. W., and Shank, J.: Student-teacher contracting: A vehicle for individualizing instruction. *Audiovisual Instruction.* *18*: 31-34, January 1973.

Several brief suggestions for design and use of grade contracts.

PROGRAMMED INSTRUCTION: OVERVIEW

DESCRIPTION Programmed Instruction (P.I.) is a term used to encompass any type of instruction which

(a) has been **derived systematically** using behavioral objectives,
(b) is divided into a series of **discrete steps** or "frames," each of which calls for **active overt response** from the learner to the critical concepts presented; and
(c) provides immediate feedback to learners regarding the adequacy of their responses.

Generally, the **process** of programming instruction involves the following steps:

1. Analyze the behaviors to be learned.
2. Analyze the entry level characteristics of the learner.
3. Determine the objectives of the instruction.
4. Write test items to measure student achievement of objectives.
5. Design self-instructional sequences to enable learners to meet each objective.
6. Try out the materials on one student at a time to observe how the materials work (DEVELOPMENTAL TEST).
7. Revise materials until developmental testing is successful without programmer intervention.
8. Test materials on larger groups of students to obtain validation data (FIELD or PILOT TEST).
9. Revise materials until adequately validated.

The **product** of this programming **process** may be any one of the following types of programs:

- Traditional Programmed Instruction (P.I.).
  - Linear programs (see page C-101).
  - Branching programs (see page C-103).

- Adjunct programs (see page C-105).

- Clinical simulations (see page C-108).

- Programmed lectures (see page C-76 in previous section).

These products or programmed materials may be displayed by:

- Books or workbooks.

- Teaching machines.

- Computer terminals (see page C-111).

- Filmstrips.

In addition, programmed materials may utilize audiovisuals such as:

- Physical models or actual equipment.
- Audiotape.
- Filmstrips or slides.
- Videotape or film.

Depending on the instructional aim and scope, programmed materials can utilize combinations of media or be combined into a

(a) **learning package**, which is a set of self-instructional materials for a single unit of instruction utilizing a variety of alternative learning modes (see page C-113), or

(b) **learning system**, which is an entire course or program composed of many self-instructional units (see page C-115).

INSTRUCTIONAL FUNCTIONS SERVED	<ul><li>Transmitting information.</li><li>Allowing students to practice behaviors.</li><li>Providing feedback on student progress.</li></ul>
ADVANTAGES	<ul><li>Allows students to progress at their own rates.</li><li>If properly tested and validated, can assure high degree of mastery for all or most students.</li><li>Frees instructor to provide individualized assistance when needed.</li><li>Provides continuous feedback to students on their learning progress.</li><li>Often saves learner's time in comparison with formal classroom instruction.</li><li>Particularly valuable when large numbers of students are involved but available in different locations and at different times.</li></ul>
LIMITATIONS	<ul><li>Generally expensive to design and validate; usually requires technical assistance from a trained programmer (i.e., an instructional technologist).</li><li>Most forms of programmed instruction are difficult to update.</li><li>Sometimes unable to maintain student motivation unless combined with other techniques specially designed to "provide a reason to learn."</li><li>Generally not appropriate for shaping attitudes or teaching complex interpersonal skills.</li></ul>

SELECTION OF PROGRAMS

Since the development of programmed materials is time-consuming, it is often advisable for instructors to utilize existing published materials rather than develop their own. The following guidelines may assist in the selection of such programs:

(a) Scan the program to determine if the **tone** and **treatment of subject** are appropriate to your instructional situation.

(b) Since self-instructional materials should be pilot-tested with a group of students, look for validation reports. These may be included with program or with an instructor's guide.

(c) Examine following information, which should be included with a carefully designed program:

- Description of the population for whom the program is intended, including prerequisites.

- List of objectives, behaviorally stated.

- A pre- and a posttest, based on the objectives.

- Description of the validation procedure including:

  - size and composition of the test group,
  - average completion times,
  - pre- and posttest scores.

REFERENCES

Becker, J. L.: *A Programmed Guide to Writing Auto Instructional Programs.* Camden, N.J.: RCA, 1963.

A programmed text on programming techniques designed for educational and industrial application.

Brethower, D. M. et al: *Programmed Learning: A Practicum.* Ann Arbor, Mich.: Ann Arbor Publishers, 1965.

A comprehensive guide to programming including chapters on subject matter analysis, frame construction, testing and revision. Most examples from industry.

Markle, S. M.: *Good Frames and Bad: A Grammar of Frame Writing.* New York: John Wiley, 1969.

An excellent programmed guide to frame writing, discussing principles of programming as well as techniques for constructing linear branching and mathematic programs.

Rowntree, D.: *Basically Branching: A Handbook for Programmers.* London: MacDonald and Co., 1966.

A readable handbook written for those who want to design branching programs. Includes a useful chapter on constructing multiple choice answer alternatives for branching programs.

Vanderschmidt, L.: Self-instructional materials for health care facilities. *Instructional Technology in Medical Education, Proceedings of the Fifth Rochester Conference on Self-Instruction in Medical Education.* Lysaught, J. (Ed). Rochester: The Rochester Clearinghouse on Self-Instruction for Health Care Facilities, 1974.

Comprehensive annotated bibliography on programmed texts, computer-aided instruction and simulation games for all categories of health professionals. Articles on self-instruction included. Validation reports cited in program description.

LINEAR PROGRAMS

DESCRIPTION
In a **linear program**, the instructional material is arranged in a series of frames forming a single uni-directional sequence. The student responds to each frame, is given immediate feedback, then advances to the next frame. A linear program could be diagrammed as follows:

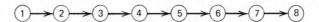

Each "balloon" represents one frame in a linear program.

ADVANTAGES
- One of the easiest types of programmed instruction both to construct and to use.
- Can give attention to fine-grain details of performance.
- When a single fixed sequence appears both optimum and reasonable for all or most of the students.

LIMITATIONS
- Difficult to use as a reference source in most cases.
- May seem tedious because of monotony of format.

The following sequence of two frames is excerpted from a program on medical interviewing.

---

1. Frequently a patient will reply to a facilitation or open-ended question with the question, "How do you mean?" The following exchange is an example.

Dr.:	Tell me about your chest pain.
Mr. Baker:	It just hurts.
Dr.:	It hurts?
Mr. Baker:	Yes!
Dr.:	Tell me about it.
Mr. Baker:	How do you mean?

   You have now used a reflection and two open-ended questions without getting a description of the pain. At this point Mr. Baker needs some support and guidance. A technique frequently used in this situation is a laundry—list question that gives the patient a number of alternative adjectives or descriptive phrases to use.

   Which of the following might be considered laundry—list question?

   A. Is it a burning pain?

   B. Does the pain go down your arm?

   C. Does the pain feel like a burn, ache, drawing, pressure, or piercing?

   D. Does it come on every week, every hour, every month or every few minutes?

   Answer: C and D.

2. Pt.: This cough is worse.
   Dr.: How is that?
   Pt.: What do you mean?

   How would you phrase a laundry-list question to learn what the patient means by "worse?"

   Answer: Compare your answer with this response: "Well, is it more frequent, deeper, productive of phlegm, making your throat sore, keeping you awake, or what?"

R.E. Froelich, and M. F. Bishop: *Medical Interviewing*. The C.V. Mosby Company, 1969.
Source. Robert E. Froelich, and Marian F. Bishop, *Medical Interviewing*, 2nd ed. St. Louis: The C. V. Mosby Co., 1972.

BRANCHING PROGRAMS

DESCRIPTION

Branching programs provide information, usually a paragraph or a group of paragraphs, and then ask students to respond to the main teaching point by way of a multiple-choice question. Three or four logical choices are provided. Depending on the student's answer, he is routed to remedial frames (if incorrect) or he advances to the next teaching point (if he is correct). A simplified diagram of a branching program looks somewhat like this:

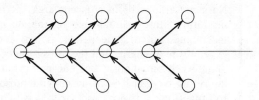

The trunk indicates the path of a student who chooses correct answers only. The branches represent wrong answer alternatives. Notice that at each branch the student is returned to the original frame before he is allowed to continue. Some branching programs, however, include sophisticated branching alternatives: for example,

- If a student misses a diagnostic question he is routed to an extensive remedial sequence.

- If a student successfully answers a question, he is asked to skip forward.

ADVANTAGES

- Can be used when students have diverse entry level competencies.

- Excellent for teaching concepts, decision-making, and problem-solving since incorrect responses normally reveal diagnosable difficulties.

- Large step size and alternative routes may make materials more attractive to persons with substantial education backgrounds.

LIMITATIONS

- Excessive page turning when presented in book form.

- Almost impossible to use as a reference.

- Not all logical incorrect answer alternatives can be conveniently included.

EXAMPLE

The following segment was taken from a program on electrocardiography:

You will probably remember that, under normal conditions, all living cells have a positive electrical charge on their surface, the inside of the cell being negative relative to the outside. Because the two sides of the cell membrane thus have polarity, like the two terminals of a battery, the cell is said to be polarized.

The reason for this electrical difference across the membrane—or MEMBRANE POTENTIAL as it is usually termed—is that the extracellular concentration of positively charged ions (cations) is somewhat higher than that inside the cell. You will also remember that the chief extracellular cation is sodium (Na+) and the chief intracellular cation is potassium (K+).

Normally, the cells in adjacent areas of tissue carry surface charges of identical magnitude. But maintenance of the unequal ionic concentrations on which the membrane potential depends is an active metabolic process, requiring the expenditure of energy and the utilisation of oxygen (the so-called "sodium pump"). Should cell metabolism become compromised, e.g. by traumatic or inflammatory injury, by oxygen lack or by enzyme poisons, the membrane will no longer be able to function actively and will have only the properties of any nonvital semipermeable membrane. Potassium will diffuse out of the cell, sodium will diffuse in; and the membrane potential will disappear.

Now decide whether the following statement is correct or incorrect: "There is no potential difference between two adjacent areas of healthy tissue in the resting state"

Correct . . . page 39   Incorrect . . . page 25

Your answer was that the statement was incorrect, or in other words, that there is a potential difference between two adjacent areas of healthy tissue. But we have already noted that healthy cells of the same tissue carry positive surface charges of identical magnitude. If the surface charges are identical, there is no potential difference between two such cells, or between two groups of cells. Only if one of the cells, or one of the groups, is damaged to the extent that it can no longer maintain the positive surface charge, will a potential difference appear. Return to page 10 and select the right answer.

Correct. There is no potential difference because cells in adjacent areas of healthy tissue normally carry identical positive charges. Now consider the two statements below. Which of these do you think is true?

Anoxic tissue is electrically positive with respect to an adjacent area of healthy tissue . . . page 9

Healthy tissue is electrically positive to an adjacent area of anoxic tissue . . . page 36

Source. S. G. Owen, *Electrocardiography, a Programmed Text*, Boston, Little, Brown & Co., 1966.

ADJUNCT PROGRAMS

DESCRIPTION

An **adjunct program** is a type of programmed instruction in which a separate "adjunct" is written to accompany another text. The adjunct contains all instructions to the students and question-answer sequences for the program, and the text contains the instructional content. The process for programming instruction is followed, but once the terminal student competencies and test items are specified, the method selected to lead students to respond appropriately to these questions differs from traditional programmed instruction in that the "adjunct" directs the learner to:

(a) read certain pages in the text; These pages may be part of:

— pre-existing books, manuals, articles, or phamphlets; or
— specially prepared handouts, books, manuals, or tables;

(b) answer one or more questions in which they are asked to respond to the most important concepts, to practice critical discriminations, and/or to apply the information read so as to meet the instructional objectives; and

(c) compare his/her own responses to the feedback provided. Learners are also encouraged to review portions of the text when they answer incorrectly and do not understand why.

ADVANTAGES

- Instructors can utilize preexisting materials and still have the advantages of individualized interactive instruction. For example, many excellent texts are available in the health fields, but they are often too tedious to maintain student motivation without periodic changes in pace or opportunity for self-testing.

- Content can be used later for **reference** purposes (unlike traditional P. I. where the content is embedded in the question sequences).

- Adjunct programs can be prepared with **less time** and resources than traditional P. I. Even if the content is not already available in an acceptable form, less time is required to organize and write prose text than is necessary for a linear or branching format.

- Adjunct programs are particularly good for advanced students who are capable of reading and digesting large segments of information.

- Students have more control over their progress than in traditional P. I. since they can

(a) read question sequences before reading the text if they prefer;
(b) read more than one segment of text at a time before answering questions on either segment;
(c) go back and review any part of the text at any point.

LIMITATIONS

- It is not as **efficient** a mode of initial instruction as traditional P. I. in that:

  (a) students usually must read more information than they must know to answer the questions, and
  (b) students must digest and interpret much of what they read without immediate feedback.

- During the initial learning process, students may find it cumbersome to alternate between the text and the adjunct itself.

- Revision on the basis of student feedback is difficult because it is hard to trace a student error to the source in the text.

EXAMPLE 1

A national pharmaceutical manufacturer wanted to be sure its salesmen had complete, current, and accurate product knowledge to present to physicians.

This product information was already available to the salesmen in the form of direction circulars, which are descriptive brochures accompanying all drugs originating from a drug manufacturer. However, since the form of this information is tightly regulated by the Food and Drug Administration, such direction circulars are difficult to read. (Even physicians have been known to refuse to read them.)

The company decided to prepare product knowledge tests for their most important products, and to require salesmen failing to achieve an acceptable score on one of these tests to work through an Adjunct to the relevant direction circular before taking the test again.

These Adjuncts consisted of booklets containing:

(a) Instructions directing the reader to specific sections of the direction circular.
(b) Review questions covering the critical points (similar to or, in some cases, duplicates of the questions asked in the formal product knowledge test).
(c) Special "teaching sequences" to provide specific medical terminology considered prerequisite to understanding the direction circular.

EXAMPLE 2

The Adult Learning Laboratory of the American College of Life Underwriters has developed several self-instructional packages to send to registrants of their correspondence courses. These packages consist of the relevant textbooks, an adjunctive Study Guide, and any other materials needed to complete the module. The Study Guide contains the following sections:

a. *Purpose and significance*—a one-page description of what the assignment is about and why it is important in relation to its eventual use.
b. *Objectives*—a listing of behaviorally-stated objectives for the assignment.

c. *Reference and questions*—directions to read portions of the textbook or to do some other learning activity, followed by questions related to a given objective.

d. *Summary*—review of relevant points and feedback to questions in Section 3.

e. *Illustrative problems*—practice problems similar to those to appear on the final examination, complete with answers.

REFERENCES

Langdon, D. G. Confirmation via/and a summary. *NSPI Journal* 1970, *9*, 7-17.

Describes the adjunctive study guide approach to college level correspondence courses now used at the Adult Learning Laboratory of the American College of Life Underwriters (270 Bryn Mawr Ave., Bryn Mawr, Pennsylvania, 19010).

Rocklyn, E. H., Sullivan, J. R. O., and Zemke, R. Olivetti programming: A useful programming variation. *Training and Development Journal*, January 1968, 40-46.

Provides guidelines for writing adjuncts to existing technical materials.

CLINICAL SIMULATIONS

DESCRIPTION

Clinical simulations, also called patient management problems, are complex branching programs that attempt to simulate clinical case situations. Clinical simulations usually consist of:

(a) brief case description listing the patient's chief complaints,
(b) multiple-choice questions asking what actions the "attending physician" should take, and
(c) feedback including remedial sequences for incorrect responses.

A clinical simulation usually begins with questions on data collection, such as "what information is needed?" and "what tests should be ordered?". Information must be collected by the learner with proper consideration for effectiveness, efficiency, and patient safety. Once the student has collected sufficient information, he evaluates it and plans effective therapy and patient management. Management, therapy, or disposition often require the physician to handle items of specialized information, some of which may be incomplete or conflicting.

Clinical simulations are often displayed by a computer but paper-and-pencil versions have also been published.

ADVANTAGES

- Approximates the physician's real-world performance.

- Can be used to teach and/or to assess complex problem-solving skills.

- Allows medical students to treat a wide variety of cases in a relaxed setting. Such problems may be selected to sample the range of behaviors that the physician should demonstrate.

- May be sequenced from simple to difficult, thus allowing the student to progress from "clean" problems to problems that include ambiguities and complex discriminations.

- Builds the following skills:

  − Facility in handling complex conflicting data.
  − Development of strategies for problem-solving.

LIMITATIONS

- Difficult to construct.

- Expensive to display via computer.

- Difficult to validate: Does skill in solving this type of problem transfer to the physician's on-the-job performance?

EXAMPLE   An example of a segment for a computer-displayed clinical simulation appears on the following page.

REFERENCES

McGuire, C. H. and Solomon, L. M.: *Clinical Simulations: Selected Problems in Patient Management.* New York: Appleton Century Crofts, 1971.

A collection of paper-and-pencil clinical simulations designed to train medical students in clinical decision-making.

Massachusetts General Hospital Laboratory of Computer Science: *Computer-Based Programs.* Boston: Harvard Medical School, 1973.

Published through the support of the National Library of Medicine, Lister Hill National Center for Biomedical Communications; provides directions for accessing 10 clinical simulations developed by the Laboratory of Computer Science on such topics as Abdominal Pain, Cardiac Simulations, Cardiopulmonary Resuscitation, Diabetic Ketoacidosis, Jaundice, etc. Sections from each program are given.

Wilds, P. L. and Zachert, V.: *Programmed Instruction in Teaching Patient Management.* Augusta, Ga.: Medical College of Georgia, 1967.

A compilation of examples of paper-and-pencil clinical simulations. Included are case presentations for teaching clinical reasoning skills, and guidelines for developing such presentations.

LET ME BRIEFLY EXPLAIN THIS PROGRAM. WE ARE GOING TO SIMULATE A RESUSCITATION. A SITUATION WILL BE PRESENTED AND YOU WILL GO STEPWISE THROUGH AN ATTEMPT AT RESUSCITATING THE PATIENT BY ANSWERING A SERIES OF MULTIPLE CHOICE QUESTIONS. DEPENDING ON WHAT YOU DO TO THE PATIENT, HIS STATUS MAY CHANGE THOUGH NOT ALWAYS AS EXPECTED (AS IN REAL LIFE.) DOING THE SAME THING TO A SIMULATED PATIENT IN APPARENTLY SIMILAR SITUATIONS MAY NOT ALWAYS HAVE THE SAME OUTCOME. OUR SETTING WILL ALWAYS BE A REGULAR FLOOR, NOT THE EW OR ICU AND YOU WILL INITIALLY BE ALONE. YOU WILL THUS NOT BE ABLE TO DO THINGS SIMULTANEOUSLY AS YOU MAY WISH.

THE PATIENT IS A 74 YEAR OLD MAN WHO IS 2 DAYS POST IRIDECTOMY. YOU ARE A STAT CONSULT BECAUSE THE PATIENT DOES NOT LOOK RIGHT.

WHAT DO YOU DO FIRST?

1. TAKE AN EKG
2. START AN IV
3. CHECK MAJOR VESSELS FOR PULSES, SEE IF PATIENT IS RESPONSIVE
4. GIVE A SHOT OF INTRACARDIAC EPINEPHRINE

>3

  PT STIRS AS YOU POKE NECK
BEING CALLED TO AN ARREST DOES NOT AUTOMATICALLY MEAN THAT ONE EXISTS; IN THIS INSTANCE THE PATIENT WAS ONLY SLEEPING

YOUR SCORE FOR THIS CASE WAS: 100

COMMENT (Y/N)? NO

THE PATIENT IS A 69 YEAR OLD MAN WHO IS CONVALESCING FROM A RECENT MI. YOU ARE TOLD THAT HE LOOKS ILL, RUSH IN AND FIND THAT HE DOES NOT SEEM TO BE BREATHING.

WHAT DO YOU DO FIRST?

1. TAKE AN EKG
2. START AN IV
3. CHECK MAJOR VESSELS FOR PULSES, SEE IF PATIENT IS RESPONSIVE
4. GIVE A SHOT OF INTRACARDIAC EPINEPHRINE

>3

THERE ARE NO PALPABLE CAROTID OR FEMORAL PULSES; THE PATIENT DOES NOT RESPOND TO YOUR SHOUT. WHAT IS YOUR NEXT MOVE?

1. START CLOSED CHEST MASSAGE
2. GIVE A SHARP BLOW TO THE PRECORDIUM WITH YOUR FIST
3. QUICKLY GO OUT AND YELL FOR HELP
4. TAKE AN EKG

>2

Laboratory of Computer Science, Massachusetts General Hospital.

COMPUTER-ASSISTED INSTRUCTION

DESCRIPTION

In **computer-assisted instruction** (CAI), information (text, questions, and diagrams) is stored in the computer and is usually displayed for the learner on a TV-like screen (cathode tube) or typed out on a computer terminal. The learner may give the computer commands or ask questions by using the typewriter keyboard and (depending on the programming) also draw (or point/choose) on the screen using a light-pen device.

Computers can be used to present linear and adjunct programs, but their advantages are better utilized by clinical simulations and other complex branching programs.

ADVANTAGES

- Convenient provision of complicated branching.

- Possibility of using prior learner responses as the basis for determining the next instructional step.

- Computers can compile data on how many students selected various incorrect responses, thus assisting in the improvement of the instructional content.

LIMITATIONS

- Cost per student hour is high in computer-assisted instruction, particularly when the computer is used as a supplement to instruction. In applications (courses) where the computer is the sole delivery instrument for instruction, its costs may be comparable to instruction delivered as effectively in other ways.

- Good software (i.e., the programs, as opposed to the computer hardware) that can be used anywhere is not yet available. Users still are writing programs that can be used on only one type of machine.

REFERENCES

Bundy, R. F.: *Bibliography on Computer-Assisted Instruction* (mimeo). Rochester, N.Y.: The Clearinghouse on Self-Instructional Materials for Health Care Facilities, University of Rochester, 1967.

Listing of approximately 170 articles and books related to computer-assisted instruction.

Computer-Assisted Instruction/Computer-Managed Instruction Information Exchange. Newburyport, Mass.: ENTELEK, Inc., updated bimonthly.

Four types of data are contained in bimonthly volumes of cards: abstracts of the CAI literature, specifications of CAI programs, abstracts of the CMI literature, and descriptions of CAI/CMI facilities. Subclassifications include the health professions, diagnosis, patient management, nursing, and dentistry.

Farquhar, J. A. et al: *Applications of Advanced Technology to Undergraduate Medical Education* (Memorandum RM-6180-NLM) Santa Monica, Cal.: The Rand Corporation, 1970.

Six examples of the application of advanced technology to medical education are described, including computer-assisted instruction and computer-assisted self-evaluation. The report includes a discussion of the impact and goals of applying technology to medical education and presents directives for future research.

Hickey, A. E.: *Computer-Assisted Instruction: A Survey of the Literature.* Newburyport, Mass.: ENTELEK, Inc., 1968.

A selective review and synthesis of over 1000 reports of research, development, and application in the field of computer-assisted instruction. Special sections include: an overview of CAI in the United States and abroad; applications in the health professions—diagnosis, patient management, nursing, and dentistry; descriptions of systems and programming languages; and a discussion of the implementation and administration of CAI.

Proceedings of the Conference on the Use of Computers in Education. Oklahoma City, Okla.: University of Oklahoma Medical Center, 1968.

A collection of papers and reports of panel discussions focusing on the current use and potentials of computers in undergraduate, clinical, and continuing medical education.

Stolurow, L. M., Peterson, T. I., and Cunningham, A. C. (Eds.): *Computer-Assisted Instruction in the Health Professions.* Newburyport, Mass.: ENTELEK, Inc., 1970.

Collection of 33 papers presented at the 1968 Conference on CAI in Medical Education sponsored by the Office of Naval Research and held at the Harvard Medical School. Reports on the application of CAI to medical, dental, and nursing education at Harvard, Ohio State, Oklahoma, the Naval Medical School, and other locations. Examines cost, effectiveness, and trends in the application of CAI in teaching surgery, anesthesia, ophthalmology, patient interviewing and management, medical records, and other topics.

LEARNING PACKAGES

DESCRIPTION

A learning package is a module or single unit that guides the individual student's learning activities in a limited subject area. Typically it contains information in these categories:

- *Overview/rationale.* *What* is to be learned and **why** it is important to the student.

- *Objectives.* One or more behaviorally stated objectives defining the scope of the activity and the desired accomplishments.

- *Resources.* The instructional/learning resources that can be used in attaining the objectives, which may include a variety of media/methods.

- *Activities.* Optional or required activities, using the resources, that are deemed appropriate for attaining the objectives.

- *Evaluation.* Explicit information describing how the work to be done will be evaluated. Learning packages may include a pretest, a prerequisite test, a self-test, and/or posttests.

Often these learning packages form the basic "building blocks" in a larger learning system. (See page C-115.)

ADVANTAGES

- Permits alternate, learner-managed paths to the same objectives.

- When used as modules in a larger learning system, can permit control over learning by requiring mastery of a unit as the condition for moving on to the next.
- Usually less expensive and time-consuming to develop than traditional programmed instruction.

- Encourages learner self-discipline and learning how to learn.

LIMITATIONS

- Requires substantial development effort in comparison with lectures.

- May result in logistic problems: ensuring adequate inventory of resources, providing evaluations when needed, etc.

REFERENCES

Jackson, P.: *Writer's LAP.* Ft. Lauderdale, Fa., Education Association Inc., 1971.

A learning package designed to teach others to develop learning packages. Intended primarily for elementary and secondary teachers, but usable by teachers in the health professions.

Johnson, R. and Johnson S: *Directory of Self Instructional Materials: Self Instructional Materials Project.* Southern Medical School Consortium, Trailer 16, Manning Drive, University of North Carolina, Chapel Hill, N.C., 27514, 1972.

Lists learning packages developed for medical school use and packages designed for allied health schools. Packages are described in terms of specialty area, author, target populations, objectives, time to complete, availability, and format.

LEARNING SYSTEMS

DESCRIPTION

A **learning system** is an assemblage of individualized instructional units predesigned to permit students to progress at their own rates to achieve stated objectives. Learning systems are not, properly speaking, an "instructional method." Rather, they are entire courses that have been programmed using a systematic approach. A learning system incorporates whatever instructional activities are available to best achieve the level of simulation required. As such, they utilize combinations of methods and media.

Characteristics of many learning systems:

- Students may be tested to determine entry-level performance, with appropriate branching provided.

- Student may select some of the topics to be studied and when to study those topics. Student may contract for particular grades by agreeing to accomplish a given number of tasks or units satisfactorily in a prespecified amount of time.

- Students work at their own pace.

- A mixture of learning activities are included, each of which aims at optimizing teacher time and student learning. These activities may consist of:

  - traditional P. I. (linear or branching)
  - adjunct programs
  - readings, such as books or articles
  - films, film strips, videotapes, audiotapes, or any multi-media combination
  - laboratory work or experiments
  - library research
  - etc.

- Learning activities are often organized by sets of required/optional "learning packages" (see page C-113). Students must demonstrate mastery of each package or module before proceeding to the next one.

- Students generally interact with an instructor, proctor, teaching assistant, or coordinator at regular intervals—but more for purposes of motivation, discussion, and feedback than for imparting content.

- Students complete the course only when they have met objectives.

ADVANTAGES

- Can provide for a wide variety of learning styles, by incorporating a broad range of learning activities from which the student may choose.

- Students proceed at their own pace, master the material thoroughly, and have the close attention of, at least, one member of the teaching staff.

- Systematic design incorporating evaluation feedback makes it possible to revise and improve the learning system or parts within the system.
- Once validated, such systems can be shared by institutions having similar student populations and educational goals.

LIMITATIONS	• Expensive to design and produce. Simply gathering the materials and organizing them into compact, self-contained units requires time and money.

- Requires faculty retraining.
- Students sometimes feel that they are being deprived when the major professor makes only a few presentations each semester.
- Some students prefer that their chief staff contact, however infrequent, is with someone with more status than a student tutor or teaching assistant.

EXAMPLE 1

Northeastern University's freshman course in psychology has been translated into a learning system. Six thousand students rotate through this system annually, 1500 per instructional quarter. The course, entitled *Interact with Psychology,* includes programmed text, articles, videotapes, films, and tests. When students take this course, they

- read preparatory programmed units,
- watch videotapes (one per week) while solving problems on worksheets provided,
- work through programmed review units,
- read articles and watch films,
- take "progress quizzes" once a week (this quiz is scored by computer and returned in two hours), and
- discuss problem areas and topics of interest in small-group sessions led by an instructor (once a week).

EXAMPLE 2

The Keller Plan, one of the first learning systems to become popular, has five basic features, as follows:

Student-paced Instruction: The basic course materials are prepared well in advance of all classes, usually in the form of printed units, which are available to students from the start of the course. Thus, one student can choose to work rapidly, finishing the work of the course by mid-semester; others may go more slowly. Many students work on the units during the appointed class hours, but each student has the option of proceeding at his own pace.

Demonstrated Mastery: Regardless of his pace, each student must demonstrate mastery of each unit by taking a short examination on that unit; if he fails, he must repeat the examination until he passes it. He may try again whenever he feels he is ready.

Prepared Study Guides: The instructor must carefully plan and prepare the study guides that form the basis of the course, gathering them into units of appropriate size, each with stated objectives, study procedures, and examination questions. These guides direct the students' learning activities; they may require reading books, watching films, listening to tapes, answering questions, etc.

Motivational Lectures: To increase the student's interest, the instructor gives occasional lectures and demonstrations that are almost solely motivational in purposes. (The transmission of information is accomplished essentially through the study guides.) Attendance at these lectures is not required and examinations are not based on them.

Student Tutors: Tutors usually are advanced students who have taken the course previously. They offer additional instruction, score examinations, and give counsel. Tutors are closer to the student in both age and experience than is the head instructor. This factor, coupled with a favorable student-tutor ratio, enable tutors to create a relationship with the student that an instructor cannot, regardless of his experience.

REFERENCES

Horn, R. E.: *Come Along with Me into My Custom Made It's Up to You Browsing Learning Growing Move Around Information Environment (If You Want To).* Lexington, Mass.: Information Resources, Inc. (P.O. Box 417), 1969.

Description of a graduate level course designed to individualize instruction. Students rotate through learning stations each of which is stocked with self-teaching materials. Students select objectives, content, sequence, and evaluation procedures.

Johnston, J. M., and Pennypacker, H. S.: A behavioral approach to college teaching. *American Psychologist. 26*: 219-244, 1971.

This paper describes in detail a Keller-type approach to teaching college psychology. It stresses the use of student managers, who are upper-level students responsible for guiding or managing the learning of lower-level students.

Keller, F. S.: Good-bye teacher, . . . *Journal of Applied Behavioral Analysis. 1*: 79-89, 1968.

The original article on the Keller Plan by the person who developed the concept.

Kulik, J. A., Kulik, C. L., and Carmichael, K.: The Keller plan in science teaching. *Science. 183*: 379-383, 1974.

This review article cites research designed to evaluate the Keller plan.

Sherman, J. G.: *PSI: Personalized System of Instruction: 41 Germinal Papers.* Menlo Park, Cal.: W. A. Benjamin, 1974.

These papers have been collected to serve as a guide for persons who wish to try the Keller Plan (PSI) in new contexts. The papers, through example, illustrate the method, research, findings, and history of PSI

MEDIA

INTRODUCTION   Media are the vehicles or channels through which information is transmitted. This section describes the most common media available to instructors for presenting auditory and/or visual information to students.

DIRECTORY

CHALKBOARD

DESCRIPTION   The chalkboard has great utility in a classroom:

(a) For presentations that are **developed** during class; for example, to illustrate the interrelationship of component parts of a subject, a sequence of events, or a trial-and-error approach to a problem.

(b) To visually present information responsive to immediate needs, that is, clarify concepts on-the-spot, or to consider questions as they come up.

(c) When changes and rearrangements of information in the presentation are needed.

(d) To record ideas contributed by different individuals on-the-spot.

(e) To present an outline or overview of the day's lecture or discussion topic.

ADVANTAGES

- Little preparation time is needed.

- Display is prepared by the instructor, who can alter it on-the-spot as appropriate.

- Simple to use and readily available in most classrooms.

- Lends itself to spontaneity while lecturing or giving demonstrations.

LIMITATIONS

- Instructor turns his back to class while writing.

- Audience size is limited.

- Dependent on instructor's graphic/writing skills.

- Presentations are not reusable unless copied before or after the class session.

- Complex or cumulative displays must be planned beforehand so relationships will be clear when the final product is viewed.

REFERENCES   Kemp, J. E.: Magnetic Chalkboards. *Planning and Producing Audiovisual Materials.* Scranton, Pa.: Chandler Publishing Co., pp 222-223, 1968.

Includes instructions for making a homemade magnetic chalkboard.

Pula, F. J.: Chalkboards. *Making Educational Communication Work.* Dubuque: Kendall/Hunt, pp. 157-158, 1972.

Describes use of templates, opaque projections, prepared patterns, grids, semipermanent displays.

Wittich, W. A. and Schuller, C. F.: The Chalkboard. *Audiovisual Materials: Their Nature and Use.* New York: Harper and Row, pp. 73-91, 1967.

Discussion of chalkboard selection and use, and drawing aids.

FLIP CHART

DESCRIPTION
A **flip chart** is a large pad of paper (approximately 2 x 3 ft) attached to a portable easel. The paper can be plain or printed with lines, grids, etc. Information is displayed by writing on the sheets with markers; or more elaborate presentations can be prepared in advance.

ADVANTAGES
- Can be used as a substitute for or supplement to the chalkboard and overhead projector.

- Easel and pads are comparatively inexpensive, convenient to store and transport.

- Can prepare charts before class and flip them over when needed.

- Permits displays to be preserved for reuse.

- Sheets can be torn off and attached to the wall to develop cumulatively related displays.

LIMITATIONS
- Storage can be a problem since pads are large.

- Generally not satisfactory for use with large audiences.

- Dependent on graphic skills of instructor (if not prepared in advance by a graphic artist).

EXAMPLE 1
Teams working on the same problem can enter their solutions on a sheet from the flip chart. Then, after all solutions have been completed, all of the team productions can be displayed side-by-side for instructor and participant comments.

EXAMPLE 2
To teach complex procedures, some instructors use two flipcharts, one for displaying each abstract step involved in the procedure, and the other for showing examples or specific applications of the steps.

OVERHEAD PROJECTION

DESCRIPTION

Overhead projection involves projecting images from a plastic "transparency" onto a projection surface such as a screen or wall.

A **transparency** is an 8 1/2 × 10 in. sheet of clear plastic that may be blank or contain prepared images.

The instructor can write directly on the transparency while the image is being projected with an overhead projector, much as one would write on a chalkboard. Prepared transparencies can be purchased ready-made or easily produced by the instructor using a variety of methods. For example, equipment is available that can produce a transparency duplicate of most printed materials.

Masking devices allow instructors to uncover a sequence of points one by one; and overlay films can be used to build complex figures in a series of small steps.

DIAGRAM

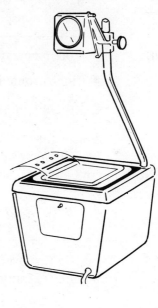

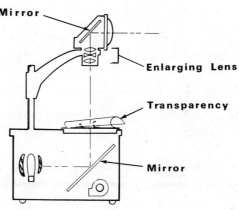

ADVANTAGES

- Transparencies are inexpensive to make and, if appropriate, can be cleaned and reused.

- Can display copies of student-generated work.

- If care is taken to prepare transparencies with large images, presentations can be made to large audiences.

- Projector is positioned at the front of the room rather than in the audience.

- Instructor has access to projector while still maintaining face-to-face contact with the audience and can see the visual while it is on the projector.

- Projector can be used under normal room-light conditions.

- Order of visual presentation can be easily altered by the presenter in response to audience reactions.

- Projector can be used with a variety of objects, besides transparencies: flat opaque objects with recognizable shapes; liquids presented in petri dishes, transparent objects such as syringes, thermometers.

LIMITATIONS

- More preparation time than with a chalkboard.

- Cumbersome to carry and use a large number of transparencies.

- Difficult to make illustrations requiring shaded areas or tones.

SOURCES OF TRANSPARENCIES

National Information Center for Educational Media (NICEM): *Index to Educational Overhead Transparencies.* Los Angeles: University of Southern California, annual.

Annotated subject and title index of commercially available transparencies, 50,000 entries.

REFERENCES

Kemp, J. E.: Overhead transparencies. *Planning and Producing Audiovisual Materials.* Scranton, Pa.: Chandler Publishing, 1968.

Describes in detail several methods of making transparencies.

Minor, E.: *Simplified Techniques for Preparing Visual Instructional Materials.* New York: McGraw-Hill, 1962.

Includes a generously illustrated chapter on preparing transparencies.

Smith, R. E.: *The Overhead System: Production Implementation and Utilization.* Austin: University of Texas, Visual Instruction Bureau, n. d.

Manual illustrating various techniques of preparing transparencies.

35MM SLIDES

DESCRIPTION

The **35mm slide** is a photographic reproduction of an image on transparent film. The image on the slide is projected onto a large screen with any 35mm projector for viewing by either small or large audiences. Thirty-five millimeter slides are produced by photographing with any 35mm camera:

(a) animate or inanimate subject matter
(b) illustrations and graphic information from books, manuals, brochures, magazines and newspapers.

DIAGRAM

35 mm Slides

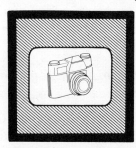

Double – Frame
Aperture dimension
23mm x 34mm

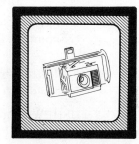

"Super" Slide
Aperture dimension
2 3/16 in. x 2 3/16 in.

ADVANTAGES

- Can reproduce for a large audience critical detailed information in its natural color or in black-and-white (e.g., X rays, visually observable signs such as a skin rash, etc).

- Instructor can use remote control mechanism to change slides while standing in front of the audience.

- Slides are reusable. They can be stored safely in trays ready for presentation, or resequenced for each new presentation.

- Equipment for preparation of slides (35mm camera) and for presentation (slide projector and screen) are comparatively inexpensive and usually readily available in instructional settings.

- Commercially prepared slide sets are available for purchase at reasonable prices.

LIMITATIONS

- Time delay for processing of film (from 3 to 10 days).

- Room must be darkened for effective presentation.

SOURCES   National Information Center for Educational Media (NICEM): *Index to Educational Slides.* Los Angeles: University of Southern California, annually.

Annotated subject and title index of commercially available educational slides, 18,000 entries.

REFERENCES   Erickson, C. W. H.: The 2-inch by 2-inch slide. *Fundamentals of Teaching with Audiovisual Technology.* New York: Macmillan, 1965.

Steps are given for making 2 in. by 2 in. slides from originals (magazines, maps, etc.) at hand.

Kemp, J. E.: Slide series. *Planning and Producing Audio-visual Materials.* Scranton, Pa.: Chandler Publishing, 1968.

Illustrated directions for making 2 in. by 2 in. slides, and a few considerations on projectors.

USHEW, Public Health Service: *Designing Good Slides.* Public Health Services Publication No. 2196. Washington, D.C.: U.S. Government Printing Office, 1971.

*Illustrated manual for **design** (not production) of 35mm slides.*

AUDIOTAPE

DESCRIPTION

Audiotape is a ribbon of cellulose-acetate film used to record voice, music, and/or other sounds. The only equipment needed in most instances is a **tape recorder**, which both records and plays back. Audiotapes are available in different sizes and lengths, including the standard reel-to-reel tapes and, more recently cassette tapes. Prerecorded tapes may be purchased or instructors can record their own presentations on blank tape with the use of a microphone that plugs directly into the tape recorder.

Audiotapes can be used for a variety of instructional activities, for example:

- Case studies in dialogue form can be presented by audiotape rather than in written form.

- Outside presentations or radio programs can be taped and played back in the classroom.

- Instructions for lab exercises can be taped and played back by individual students when needed.

- Student interviews can be taped and played back for critique.

- Whole lectures can be taped and made available to students for review or make-up sessions.

ADVANTAGES

- Accurate and portable reproduction of audio material.

- Easy to use and store tapes.

- Relatively inexpensive.

LIMITATIONS

- Cassette tape recordings can generally be used only with small groups. (Reel-to-reel recordings played on high quality equipment can be used for any size group.)

- Reel-to-reel tapes can be stretched or broken if not handled carefully.

- Fidelity of cassette tapes is often not of high quality. (Fidelity on reel-to-reel tapes is much better.)

FILMSTRIPS

DESCRIPTION

Filmstrips are strips of film, on which are imprinted a series of color or black-and-white photographs in a fixed sequence. Filmstrips are projected onto a screen with a filmstrip projector. The photograph appears on the screen much like a series of slides.

A filmstrip presentation is usually synchronized with sound in the form of audiotape, a record, or simply a script to be read.

DIAGRAM

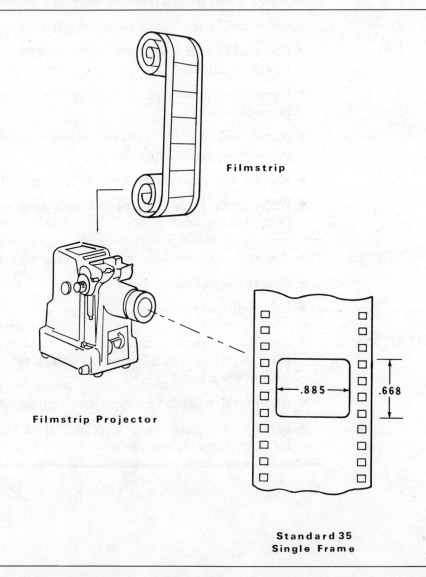

Filmstrip

Filmstrip Projector

.885 .668

Standard 35
Single Frame

ADVANTAGES

- When the same presentation is given repeatedly in the same sequence, filmstrips are less expensive and easier to store than individual slides or transparencies.

- Lends itself for both individualized and large-group viewing.

- Can be looked at under normal room light conditions as well as in specially darkened areas.

- Images can be directed on a regular projection screen or on such surfaces as a chalkboard where additional information can be set forth by the instructor.

- Depending on the size of the lamp in the projector, the filmstrip can be used effectively for groups ranging from 5 to 500.

LIMITATIONS

- Require considerable planning and production time.

- Cannot change sequence of presentation with ease.

- Cannot update presentation without preparing new filmstrip.

- Easily damaged and difficult to repair.

SOURCES

National Information Center for Educational Media (NICEM): *Index to 35mm Filmstrips.* Los Angeles: University of Southern California, annually.

Annotated subject and title index of commercially available educational filmstrips—52,000 entries.

REFERENCES

Brown, J. W., and Lewis, R. B.: *AV Instructional Materials Manual.* New York: McGraw-Hill, 1969.

Includes a section on the operation and care of filmstrip projectors.

Kemp, J. E.: Filmstrips. *Planning and Producing Audiovisual Materials.* Scranton, Pa.: Chandler Publishing, 1968.

Instructions for making one's own filmstrips, directly and from slides, illustrations and photographs.

MOTION PICTURES: 16MM FILM

DESCRIPTION Motion picture film consists of a long strip of film on which is printed a series of progressively different transparent positive images. This film, the width of which is 16 millimeters, is stored on a reel that is then mounted on a 16mm film projector. The film is pulled off the reel at a constant speed, passes through the projection system, and finally is wound onto an empty reel. The viewer sees a single image that appears to move as in real life. The length of a reel of film varies from 5 minutes to approximately 50 minutes.

DIAGRAM

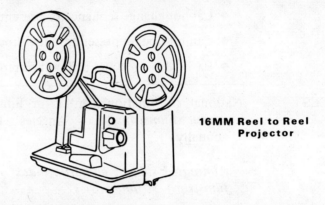

16MM Reel to Reel Projector

ADVANTAGES
- Can reproduce in the classroom the action, sound, and color of live events that have occurred elsewhere.

- Can be used for a variety of instructional functions including:

  – providing a frame of reference
  – providing a reason to learn
  – shaping student attitudes (through models)
  – demonstrating behaviors to be learned, and
  – transmitting information.

- Projection equipment is readily available and simple to operate.

- Allows for stopping and slowing down action.

- Can be shown to small or large audiences.

- A variety of 16mm films are available in the health fields that may be rented from film libraries at a reasonable cost.

LIMITATIONS
- Difficult for instructor to interject a point or idea until the end.

- Instructor loses eye contact with students, since room must be darkened for showing film.

- Expensive to produce, since both cameras and film are expensive and professional help is generally necessary.

SOURCES OF FILMS

Federal Advisory Council on Medical Training Aids: *Film Reference Guide for Medicine and Allied Sciences.* Atlanta, Ga.: National Medical Audiovisual Center, National Library of Medicine, annually.

Annotated directory of selected films used in biomedical education. Subject and title indexes.

National Information Center for Educational Media (NICEM): *Index to 16mm Educational Films.* Los Angeles: University of Southern California, annually.

Annotated subject and title index of commercially available educational films, in three volumes.

REFERENCES

Eastman Kodak Company: *Basic Production Techniques for Motion Pictures.* Rochester, New York: Eastman Kodak Co., 1971.

Short illustrated manual of 16mm film planning, production, and editing.

Kemp, J. E.: Motion pictures. *Planning and Producing Audiovisual Materials.* Scranton, Pa.: Chandler Publishing, 1968.

Background information on camera operation and sections on shooting techniques and strategies, editing, and sound techniques.

Pincus, E.: *Guide to Filmmaking.* Chicago: Henry Regnery Co., 1972.

An overall manual of filmmaking techniques, covering selection and use of equipment, production, editing, etc. For use with both 16mm and 8mm filming.

MOTION PICTURES: SUPER EIGHT-MM FILM

INTRODUCTION   Super eight-millimeter film has supplanted 16mm film as the vehicle for local film production. The lower cost of the film and equipment is both the cause and effect of this shift.

DESCRIPTION   Super 8mm film is 8mm wide and usually comes in 50-ft reels which produce approximately 3 1/2 minutes of film time. There are two ways super 8mm film can be packaged:

1. *Individual reels*—wound on a single reel and used reel-to-reel as described for 16mm films.
2. *Film cartridges* (or film loops)—encased in a plastic cartridge, the end of the film is joined to the beginning of the film in an endless loop. The film unwinds from the center and winds itself on the outside loop. No threading of film is required. The cartridge is inserted into the projector, the switch turned on, and a motion picture is immediately projected on the screen.

There are two types of projection equipment for 8mm films, for cartridge and reel-to-reel projection respectively. Cartridges operate on the same principle as the cassette tape for the cassette tape recorder. They offer such advantages as compactness, simplicity of use and protection of film.

DIAGRAM

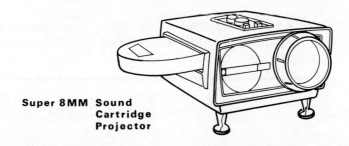

Super 8MM Sound Cartridge Projector

ADVANTAGES
- First four advantages listed for 16mm film on page C-130 apply to 8mm film as well.
- Film can be produced locally if "professional" requirements are waived, since both cameras and film are relatively inexpensive.
- 8mm film loops are effective for individual as well as group viewing. Film loops can be combined with programmed text or audiotaped presentations.

LIMITATIONS
- Smaller projected image of lesser quality than 16mm film, which tends to limit audience size.
- Few off-the-shelf 8mm films are available commercially.

- Planning and producing film is time consuming even if professional help is obtained.

- Adding sound is an independent process in most systems.

- Can't be duplicated satisfactorily.

SOURCES OF FILMS

Benschater, R. (Ed.): *8mm Films in Medicine and Health Sciences.* Lincoln, Neb.: University of Nebraska, Communications Division, 1971.

Annotated directory of 8mm films available, with subject and title listings. Includes also an annotated bibliography on production and use of 8mm films in biomedical sciences.

National Information Center for Educational Media (NICEM): *Index to 8mm Motion Cartridges.* Los Angeles: University of Southern California, annually.

Annotated subject and title index of commercially available educational films.

REFERENCES

Kemp, J. E.: Motion Pictures. *Planning and Producing Audio-visual Materials.* Scranton, Penn.: Chandler Publishing, 1968.

Background information on camera operation, and sections on shooting techniques and strategies, editing, and sound techniques.

Pincus, E.: *Guide to Filmmaking.* Chicago: Henry Regnery Co., 1972.

An overall manual of filmmaking techniques, covering selection and use of equipment, production, editing, etc. For use with both 8mm and 16mm filming.

VIDEOTAPE RECORDINGS

DESCRIPTION

Videotape records both sound and images on magnetic tape. The process requires the use of a television camera, which picks up the image through its lens system, and a tape recorder, which magnetizes the videotape as it passes the recording area. When the tape is rewound and played back through the same recorder, the image and sound are recreated on a television set (i.e., monitor) that is wired to the tape recorder.

The principle of videotape recording is basically the same as that for audiotape recording, but more complex. Video tapes are available for color, and black-and-white recording.

The most basic equipment necessary is the **tape deck**. Like an audiotape recorder, it records, plays back, rewinds and advances the tape. Tape decks vary in size, power input, and accessories, but the most important differences are the tape width, the recording speeds, the reel capacity, and whether it has color capabilities.

Other equipment needed for a videotape system include:

(a) *a camera*—available with black-and-white and/or color capacities;
(b) *a microphone*—for recording the sound portion of a videotape recording;
(c) *a TV monitor*—for displaying information recorded on the tape both while it is being recorded **and** when it is played back. (See diagram below.)

A portable tape deck and camera ensemble, referred to as the Porta-Pak, is designed for easy carrying and recording. Weighing as little as 20 pounds, it is battery-operated and has the capability of recording sound.

DIAGRAM

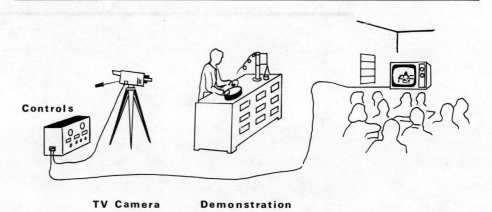

Controls

TV Camera   Demonstration

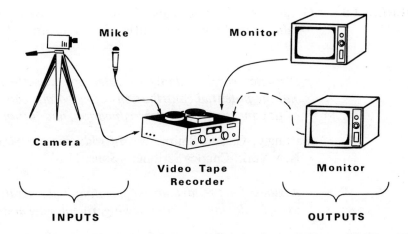

Mike   Monitor

Camera

Video Tape
Recorder

Monitor

INPUTS   OUTPUTS

ADVANTAGES

- Can be used to give students feedback on interactive events (such as patient interviews or team participation).

- Can be used to demonstrate a medical procedure (operation, workup, etc.) which should be viewed by a large group of students either while the procedure is going on or at a later time.

- Recordings can be made anywhere through the use of portable equipment.

- Immediate replay is possible, thus facilitating feedback and revision.

- Can either save presentations for later viewing or reuse the tape.

- Since sound is recorded on the tape as the picture is being recorded, no additional processing is required here.

LIMITATIONS

- Equipment is costly to buy and repair.

- Usually requires professional production staff.

- Although there is some standardization in tapes, the variety in recording systems frequently results in an incompatibility between a commercially bought tape and one's recording system.

- Bulkiness of equipment except for portable equipment.

- Harder to edit than film.

- For large audience many monitors are needed.

SOURCES

National Information Center for Educational Media (NICEM): *Index to Educational Video Tapes.* Los Angeles: University of Southern California, annually.

Annotated subject and title index of commercially available educational videotapes.

REFERENCES   Gordon, G. N. and Falk, I. A.: *Videocassette Technology in American Education.* Englewood Cliffs, N.J.: Educational Technology Publications, 1972.

Discusses current status of videotape cassette technology to education, and the potential contributions of videotape cassettes to special education, adult education, secondary education, and informal education.

Mattingly, G. and Smith, W.: *Introducing the Single-Camera VTR System.* New York: Charles Scribner's Sons, 1973.

A guide for the layman on selecting and operating videotape equipment; use of videotape in interviewing, roleplaying activities, and microteaching.

Quinn, S. F. (Ed.): *Video Cartridge, Cassette and Disc Player Systems.* Proceedings of the symposium, Oct. 7 and 8, 1971, Montreal. New York: Society of Motion Picture and Television Engineers, 1972.

A collection of papers on the state-of-the-art of videocassette technology and its applications.

REFERENCES

Regarding Media Selection

Allen, W. H.: What do fifty years of media research tell us? *Audiovisual Instruction. 18*: 48-49, March 1973.

Brief statement outlining past research (from an emphasis on "justifying" media use, to media in the learning process), and suggesting topics for further study.

Briggs, L. J., Campeau, P. L., Gagne, R. M., and May, M. A.: *Instructional Media: A Procedure for the Design of Multi-Media Instruction, A Critical Review of Research, and Suggestions for Future Research.* Pittsburgh: American Institutes for Research, 1967.

A collection of papers addressing current problems in media selection. Advances a rationale for selection based on identification of educational objectives, and on learning conditions as presented by Gagne. Includes a review of the literature by Campeau, with a critique of the shortcomings of current research. Comparative effectiveness studies, utilization studies, and basic studies are reviewed for TV, motion picture, programmed instruction, pictorial presentations, radio, recordings, three-dimensional models, and field trips. Also includes a discussion of the types of research still needed.

Gerlach, V. S. and Ely, D. P.: *Teaching and Media: A Systematic Approach.* Englewood Cliffs, N.J.: Prentice-Hall, 1971.

Chapter on media selection discusses the properties of instructional media (fixative, manipulative, distributive); the types of media; and general criteria for selection (appropriateness, level of sophistication, availability, cost, technical quality); with examples of use. A reference chapter providing specific information on 10 different types of media.

Saettler, P.: Design and selection factors. *Review of Educational Research. 38:* 115-128, April 1968. (Special issue on "Instructional Materials: Educational Media and Technology.")

Review of literature, historical overview, and a look at work done on some theoretical considerations such as multimedia design, multiple versus single-channel research, psycholinguistics of media, and communication theory.

Tickton, S. O.: *To Improve Learning. An Evaluation of Instructional Technology.* New York: R. R. Bowker Co., Vol. I, 1970.

Includes 22 "state-of-the-art" essays discussing developments in different media and their educational implications.

Tosti, D. T., and Ball, J. R.: A behavioral approach to instructional design and media selection. *AV Communication Review. 17*: 2-25, Spring 1969.

Presents a scheme for assessing media in terms of "presentation factors" inherent in the media, not the media themselves. That is, media may consist of verbal or pictorial presentation; this presentation may be transient or persistent; etc. Several such dimensions are discussed.

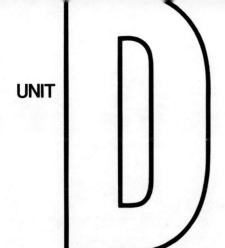

UNIT

Supplements

Unit D
SUPPLEMENTS

INTRODUCTION Unit D provides summaries of the course design model and reference aids.

Chapter 10   compiles the Guideline System as one continuous unit.
Chapter 11   compiles the same example as one continuous unit.

Chapter 10
GUIDANCE SYSTEM

The complete Guidance System is compiled here as one continuous unit. The Guidance System summarizes each major task described in Unit A, to serve as a checklist or guide when designing a course.

GUIDANCE SYSTEM

PHASE 1: DESCRIBING PROFESSIONAL PERFORMANCE

Task 1: Describe Optimal Professional Performance

STEPS	PROCEDURES	PRODUCTS
1. Identify the future professional roles of the students.	a. Indicate the future positions or titles to be assumed by students and for which training is designed. b. If future roles are widely divergent or unknown, review Problem 1 beginning on page B-6.	A phrase describing the future role(s) of the students, including information about the setting or environment in which they will practice.
2. List professional responsibilities associated with the future roles.	a. Identify the activities, duties or tasks of competent practitioners in the role(s) identified. Each activity should: — represent optimal professional performance, and — be related to the scope and purpose of the course. b. If you have difficulty with this step, consult Problems 2 and 3 in Unit B, beginning on page B-12.	A list of responsibilities for each role, organized sequentially and/or by meaningful categories.
3. Analyze the skill, knowledge, and attitude components of each responsibility.	For each responsibility: a. identify the *skills* or steps required to execute that responsibility, b. list information the practitioner must *know* or be aware of to execute a skill component or the responsibility as a whole, and c. indicate *attitudes* practitioners should have towards others, themselves, or their work to facilitate execution of a skill component or the responsibility as a whole. If you have difficulty with this step, consult Problems 4 and 5 in Unit B, beginning on page B-36.	*Initial mastery description— The complete set of professional responsibilities analyzed in terms of skill, knowledge, and attitude components. The following page shows alternative formats for these analyzed responsibilities.

*Needed in subsequent steps of the course design model.

Guidance System, continued

SUGGESTED FORMATS

For Each Analyzed Responsibility in the Mastery Description

Course Title: _____

ANALYZED RESPONSIBILITY

Responsibility No.   : _____

SKILLS	KNOWLEDGE	ATTITUDES
1. _____	_____	_____
2. _____	_____	_____
3. _____	_____	_____

OR

Course Title: _____

ANALYZED RESPONSIBILITY

Responsibility No.   : _____

A. SKILLS
   1. _____
   2. _____
   3. _____

B. KNOWLEDGE
   1. _____
   2. _____
   3. _____

C. ATTITUDES
   1. _____
   2. _____

PHASE 1: DESCRIBING PROFESSIONAL PERFORMANCE

Task 2: Analyze Actual Professional Performance

STEPS	PROCEDURES	PRODUCTS

1. Select and implement method(s) of performance analysis.	a. Review methods of performance analysis in Chapter 7, beginning on page C-3 and guidelines for selection on page B-55.
	
	b. Consider feasibility of implementation in view of constraints such as the availability of:
	
	  – time
	  – money
	  – practitioners or other subject matter experts, and
	  – resources needed to analyze data.
	
	c. Plan and carry out performance analysis.
		Instruments used in the performance analysis, such as:
		
		– questionnaires
		– checklists
		– questions for interviews
		– audio tapes for recording technical conferences

2. Identify performance discrepancies.	a. Compare findings of performance analysis with initial mastery description.
	
	b. Look for:
	
	  – responsibilities or components specified in initial mastery description which in actual practice are
	
	    • performed differently
	    • not performed well, or
	    • not performed at all.
	
	  – responsibilities or components which are performed in actual practice but were omitted from initial mastery description.
		*List of performance discrepancies.

*Needed in subsequent steps of the course design model.

GUIDANCE SYSTEM

PHASE 1: DESCRIBING PROFESSIONAL PERFORMANCE

Task 3: Revise the Initial Description of Performance

STEPS	PROCEDURES		PRODUCTS
1. Analyze causes of performance discrepancies.	Determine to what extent each discrepancy can be attributed to: — skill/knowledge factors — attitudinal factors — environmental factors.		Explanations for each performance discrepancy.
2. Modify initial mastery description.	If a discrepancy is attributed primarily to: Skill/knowledge factors Attitudinal factors Environmental factors	Then consider: → Adding or emphasizing a responsibility or appropriate skill/knowledge components. → Adding or emphasizing an attitude component to appropriate responsibilities. → Discarding the responsibility or component, or Retaining the responsibility but adding environmental constraints as knowledge components.	*Revised mastery description, which may be either — the initial mastery description which has been changed by additions, subtractions, and modifications, or — a totally new mastery description

*Needed in subsequent steps of the course design model.

GUIDANCE SYSTEM

PHASE 2: DESCRIBING STUDENT COMPETENCIES

STEPS	PROCEDURES	PRODUCTS
1. Describe professional conditions performance.	For each responsibility for which instruction is to be planned, summarize: a. typical **conditions** under which the responsibility is executed in the professional setting, and b. the **performance** of a competent practitioner discharging the responsibility under those conditions.	Descriptions of the **professional competencies** associated with each responsibility to be taught.
2. Plan simulation of the professional conditions and performance.	Determine **feasible** and **assessible** conditions and performance that most closely approximate the professional conditions and performance. Take into consideration: a. the entry competencies of the students, b. resources available for simulation, and c. needs for formal evaluation (i.e., posttests, pretests, and/or prerequisite tests). If you have difficulty with this step, consult Problems 9 to 11 in Unit B beginning on page B-70. Also, consult Chapter 8 in Unit C for details on specific evaluation techniques and related issues (page C-29).	*Descriptions of *entry* and **terminal student competencies** for each professional competency. The following page shows a suggested format for displaying these competencies.

*Needed in subsequent steps of the course design model.

Guidance System, continued

SUGGESTED FORMAT

For Describing Student Competencies

	Course Title:_____
PROFESSIONAL, TERMINAL, AND ENTRY COMPETENCIES	
Responsibility No. : _____	
CONDITIONS	PERFORMANCE
Professional Competency: When given _____ ...	.... practitioners _____ .
Terminal Student Competency: When given _____ ...	... students will _____ .
Entry Student Competencies: When given: ... (a) ... _____ ... (b) ... _____ ...	Students will ... ... _____ . ... _____ .

GUIDANCE SYSTEM

PHASE 3:   PLANNING STUDENT LEARNING

TASKS	PROCEDURES	PRODUCTS
1. Define intermediate competencies.	For each unit of instruction, specify the **conditions** and **performance** of intermediate levels of simulation for assessing student progress and providing feedback. That is, for each responsibility, determine: a. at what intermediate levels of simulation it is desirable and feasible to check student's mastery of the **entire responsibility**, and b. which skill, knowledge, and/or attitude **components** should be mastered before higher levels of simulation are attempted. For additional guidelines, see page B-100 (Problem 12 in Unit B).	Descriptions of the intermediate competencies for each terminal competency. That is, statements of the conditions and performance for intermediate levels of simulation **above** that of entry, and **below** that of the terminal competency. See following page for suggested format.
2. Design instructional activities.	a. For each unit of instruction, put intermediate competencies in an approximate sequence for instruction. b. For each intermediate competency, determine what instructional **functions** are needed to facilitate student progress from entry to termination. c. Plan activities to serve appropriate instructional functions, making sure all relevant skill, knowledge, and attitudes are covered. d. If needed, review methods and media in Chapter 9 (page C-54) and guidelines for Problems 13 and 14 in Unit B (pages B-113 and B-130).	Descriptions of instructional activities for each intermediate (and terminal) competency. Should be organized into "units of instruction." See following page for suggested format.
3. Develop course syllabus.	a. Determine final sequence for units of instruction and activities within units. b. Plan activities for continuity between units. c. Identify "assignments" to be done outside the instructional setting. d. Combine and structure in-class and out-of-class activities into the time-frame allotted for the course. e. See page B-137 (Problem 15) for additional guide-lines.	Course syllabus The following page shows a suggested format for the course syllabus.

SUGGESTED FORMATS

Course Title:_____

INTERMEDIATE COMPETENCIES

Responsibility No.   :_____

CONDITIONS	PERFORMANCE
When given . . .	Students will . . .
(Regarding Entire Responsibility:)	
1. . . ._____. . .	. . ._____.
2. . . ._____. . .	. . ._____.
(Regarding Isolated Components:)	
3. . . ._____. . .	. . ._____
4. . . ._____. . .	. . ._____
5. . . ._____. . .	. ._____
. ._____. . .	

Course Title:_____

INSTRUCTIONAL UNIT

Responsibility No.   :_____

COMPETENCIES	INSTRUCTIONAL ACTIVITIES
(Introduction to unit)	_____ _____
IC No. -	_____ _____
IC No. -	_____ _____
Terminal	_____ _____

SUGGESTED FORMATS, CONTINUED

	SYLLABUS	
Course Title: _____		Institution: _____
Unit Title: _____		Dates: _____
Date or Session	Instructional Activities	Assignments (Next Session)

Chapter 11
A COMPLETE EXAMPLE

This chapter compiles as one continuous example the major products from each phase of the course design model for a single unit of instruction.

Contents

INSTRUCTIONAL SITUATION

TITLE Pediatric Paramedical Care

PURPOSE To enable participants to care for the needs of pediatric patients presenting with the most common complaints encountered in an outpatient setting, either

  (a) by providing treatment themselves, or
  (b) by referring the case to a physician and arranging ancillary data collection if appropriate.

STUDENTS Registered nurses with at least two years of nursing experience, who have elected to become paramedics

SETTING Lashley University Medical Center in New York City

RESOURCES Sufficient funds are available to cover the costs of all necessary materials including reprints, slides, videotapes, and so on. The instructor is available to spend full-time on this course. Other full-time instructors, pediatric residents and interns, a pediatric nutritionist, and a social worker could be made available for short periods of time, but not for major teaching responsibilities. Classrooms are fully equipped with audiovisual equipment, and outpatient examining rooms are available for labs at least one day a week. A well-equipped lab where routine urine and hematology work could be performed is also accessible.

CONSTRAINTS Course begins in six months and must conform to dates established by the regular school semester at Lashley University. This schedule allows for two 2-hour class sessions and one 3-hour lab period each week for 30 weeks, or a total of 210 class hours for the year. For each class hour, students can be expected to spend between 1 and 2 hours outside of class working on assignments. Up to 20 students will take the course each year, and they must be prepared to pass certification requirements by the end of the year.

LIST OF PROFESSIONAL RESPONSIBILITIES

A pediatric paramedic . . .

*1. Takes a complete medical history from parent when appropriate.
2. Performs a complete pediatric physical examination when appropriate.
3. Performs abbreviated physical exams when needed.
4. Performs or arranges for pertinent laboratory and diagnostic tests.
5. Refers child to physician if necessary, providing appropriate clinical notes as well as test findings.
6. Provides treatment and follow-up care for each of the following types of problems:

   (a) Gastroenteritis (vomiting, diarrhea, etc).
   (b) Simple acute upper respiratory infections (e.g., colds, otitis media, pharyngitis, etc).
   (c) Simple dermatitis (impetigo, mild eczema, acne, etc).
   (d) Most nutritional problems (obesity, feeding problems, etc).
   (e) Immunizations.

7. Provides the ongoing health educational aspects of the following types of problems (in conjunction with physician care);

   (a) Behavior problems (e.g., enuresis, hyperactivity, sleep phobia, thumb sucking, etc).
   (b) Chronic diseases (e.g., diabetes mellitis, asthma, etc).
   (c) Adolescent problems (e.g., pregnancy, V.D., drugs, etc).

8. Arranges for social service referrals if appropriate (e.g., for cases of child battery, lead poisoning, etc).
9. Maintains clinical records in a problem-oriented fashion.

*This first responsibility forms the basis of the instructional unit developed in the remainder of this example.

ANALYZED RESPONSIBILITY

Responsibility No. 1: Takes a complete medical history from parent when appropriate.

SKILLS	KNOWLEDGE	ATTITUDES
1. Recognizes when a complete history is necessary.	– Complete history necessary in initial, nonemergency visit.	
2. Puts parent and patient at ease.	– Factors often making patients uncomfortable and ways to avoid them.	– Sympathetic to discomfort of the patient.
3. Determines history details using directed but nonleading questions:	– Difference between leading and non-leading questions, and between directed and non-directed questions.	– Desire to make medical history non-threatening to parent.
Chief complaint including age (accurate in months), race, and sex		
Present illness including signs and symptoms, and duration of each	– Associated signs and symptoms pertinent to each sign and symptom.	
Birth history including birth weight; age, gravity, parity, and abortions of mother; length of gestation; neonatal problems and feeding habits.	– Definitions of gravity, parity, abortion, gestation, neonatal problems to watch for.	– Senses importance of thoroughness and accuracy in taking histories.
Past history including previous hospitalizations, serious accidents or illnesses, communicable diseases, immunizations and developmental milestones	– Standard immunization routine – Common communicable diseases – Normal neonatal developmental milestones.	– Is honest in recording even those statements from parents that appear contradictory or irrelevant.
Family history including three generations whenever possible, and general health of each member	– Method for plotting family tree by age, appropriate illness, and deaths.	
Social history including type of house, number of people living in house, occupation of parents, nature of parents' relationship to child		
Review of systems including respiratory otolaryngeal, cardiovascular, gastrointestinal, genitourinary, endocrine, neurologic, and bones-joints-muscles.	– Specific questions to ask related to each system.	
4. Records history details on history form.	– Appropriate formats for each type of history data.	– Strives for legibility, clarity, and completeness when recording history details.

PROFESSIONAL, TERMINAL, AND ENTRY STUDENT COMPETENCIES

Responsibility No. 1: Takes a complete medical history from parent when appropriate.

CONDITIONS	PERFORMANCE
Professional Competency:	
When given a variety of pediatric cases in a clinical setting, history forms, and any needed decision guides	. . . practitioners determine when complete medical histories are needed, put patients and parents at ease, take histories, and record data on history forms.
Terminal Student Competency:	
When given a fellow student who has been primed with a patient scenario in a classroom setting, a history form and any needed decision guides . . .	. . . students will put the "parent" at ease, take a complete medical history, and record the data on the history form.
Entry Student Competencies:	
When given . . .	Students will . . .
(a) . . . a list of common signs and symptoms	. . . give common-sense definitions or explanations of 75% of the terms.
(b) . . . a list of organ systems and a randomized list of the different parts within these systems	. . . match parts to system in which they belong with 80% accuracy.
(c) multiple-choice questions related to: — the basic disease process — gestation periods — abortions, etc . . .	. . . select correct answers in 75% of the cases.

INTERMEDIATE COMPETENCIES

Responsibility No. 1: Takes a complete medical history from parent when appropriate.

CONDITIONS	PERFORMANCE
When given ...	Students will ...

(Regarding Entire Responsibility:)

CONDITIONS	PERFORMANCE
1. An audiotaped interview with the parent of a sick child; history form; access to decision guides	. . . record the complete medical history on the history form.
2. Incomplete case histories; access to decision flow-charts	. . . indicate what additional information is needed and why.

(Regarding Isolated Components:)

CONDITIONS	PERFORMANCE
3. a. List of common chief complaints (e.g., baby has a cold; baby not eating, etc.); plus access to decision flow charts	. . . list a question series to explore each chief complaint, excluding any factors not directly related to the chief complaint.
b. Additional history data about the patient (e.g., 3-month-old white male baby born premature)	. . . list additional questions that should be asked in light of the additional information.
4. Directions. . . .	. . . reconstruct from memory the standard immunization routine.
5. A list of most important developmental milestones plus other attained skills not considered standard neonatal milestones. . . .	. . . indicate (a) which are important neonatal milestones, and (b) give appropriate age for achieving each of these milestones.
6. A list of all persons and pertinent diseases in three generations of a family. . . .	. . . construct a medical family tree.
7. Brief descriptions of social history for particular cases. . . .	. . . indicate special diagnostic considerations and implications for therapy and patient compliance.
8. A list of general organ systems. . . .	. . . list common complaints involving each of these systems.
9. Multiple-choice questions. . . .	. . . recognize: — when a complete history is needed; — leading and nonleading questions — definitions of gravity, parity, gestation, etc. — importance of birth history, family history, etc.

INSTRUCTIONAL UNIT

Responsibility: Takes a complete medical history from parent when appropriate.

COMPETENCIES	INSTRUCTIONAL ACTIVITIES
1. (Introduction to the unit of instruction)	— Have students examine a completed history form and try to determine what the advantages of using such a form might be. — Show videotaped demonstration of complete history-taking interview, using the same case material as shown on the completed history form examined above.
*IC # 5 Given list of *milestones*, students will identify the most important and give ages for achievement.	— Have students read handout on growth and development. — Orally review the most important milestones to be memorized for convenience. — Explain the Denver Developmental Aptitude Test. — Have students list appropriate milestones for a list of given ages.
IC # 4 Students will reconstruct from memory the standard *immunization routine*.	— Have students read a handout that includes presentation and explanation of standard immunization routine. — Orally review immunization schedule, pointing out convenience of committing it to memory. — Have students practice recalling the immunization routine.
IC # 6 Given three generations of a case family, students will construct a *medical family tree*.	— Show family tree on completed history form and explain symbols; ask students about potential importance of family tree. — Using guidesheet, demonstrate construction of family tree for student volunteer. — Have students practice constructing trees and comparing results on blackboard.

*"IC # 5" means "the fifth intermediate competency listed on page A-54. Notice that the instructor has revised the order of the competencies for teaching purposes.

COMPETENCIES	INSTRUCTIONAL ACTIVITIES
IC # 7 Given cases of *social histories,* students will indicate special diagnostic considerations and implications for therapy and patient compliance.	— Have students read handout describing how to take a social history, and implications of particular types of responses. — Have students discuss possible diagnostic considerations and implications of particular social case histories.
IC # 9 Given multiple-choice items, students will recognize: — when a complete history is necessary, — leading and nonleading questions, — definitions of gravity, parity, gestation, etc. — importance of birth history, family history, etc.	— In a class discussion, have students figure out what types of visits do and do not require a complete history. — In discussion, have students practice recognizing differences between leading and nonleading questions and explain why it matters. — Have students read handout giving these definitions, and review them as they come up during class. — Have students read handout describing questions to ask in taking each part of the history, and implications of usual types of answers to questions. — In class discussion, have students determine importance of each type of question and why it needs to be asked.
IC # 8 Given list of general *organ systems,* students will list common complaints involved in each system.	— Have students read handout describing common complaints involving each organ system as well as the specific questions to be asked to elicit problems related to the systems. — Review handout stressing importance of organ systems review in subsequent visits.
IC # 3 Given *common chief complaints,* students will list question series to explore complaint, and then, on being given additional history data, will list additional questions that should be asked in light of the new data.	— Have students study a set of decision flow charts giving what questions to ask in exploring details of common chief complaints. — Demonstrate use of decision flowcharts. — Have students practice exploring chief complaints using the flowcharts (in pairs, one student primed with patient scenario). — Have students practice using the charts to list appropriate question series for particular chief complaints plus some additional case history data.

(Instructional Unit, continued)

COMPETENCIES	INSTRUCTIONAL ACTIVITIES
IC # 1 Given audiotaped interview with parent of sick child, students will record history data on a history form.	— Have students read handout listing specific questions to be asked in taking a history, how to ask and rephrase these questions, and how to record the responses onto the history form. — Demonstrate process of recording interview responses on history form. — Have students practice recording histories from audiotaped patient interviews.
IC # 2 Given incomplete case histories, students will indicate what additional information is needed and explain why it is important.	— After limited practice recording case histories as above, have students analyze incomplete case history forms, and determine what additional questions should have been asked. — In small groups, have students discuss the incomplete histories analyzed independently above.
Terminal Competency Given a classmate primed with a patient scenario, students will take a complete medical history on the history form.	— In groups of three and then in pairs, have students practice taking histories on classmates primed with scenarios. Have interviews tape-recorded and on replay, have other students give feedback before instructor comments. — Have students practice taking complete histories from actual patients under supervision of an intern or resident.

PARTIAL SYLLABUS

Course Title: Pediatric Paramedical Care

Lashley University

Unit Title: Taking Medical Histories

1974-1975

Date	Instructional Activities	Assignment for Next Session
Session 1 Sept. 24 (2 hr)	**— Introduction to Course**: Student introductions, review of syllabus, administrative details, etc. **— Instructor-led Discussion**: Major features, role, and importance of history form (centered on blank copy of form plus filled-in model form). **— Videotaped Demonstration**: Complete parent interview (same as model case). **— Instructor-led Discussion**: Of videotape, appropriate occasions for complete history, getting started (putting patient at ease, etc.)	Read **Handout A** (on growth and development, including Denver Developmental Aptitude Test).
Session 2 Sept. 26 (2 hr)	**— Mini-lecture**: Review Handout A pointing out aspects to commit to memory for convenience; explain DDAT; walk students through Handout B explaining important aspects. **— Instructor-led discussion**: Interview techniques (direct questioning; leading versus nonleading questions, etc). **— Exercise**: Have students practice recalling milestones and immunization routine. Discussion results immediately in class.	Study **Handout B** (a listing of questions to be asked for each category of history form, how to ask and rephrase these questions, important definitions, how to record responses, and explanations of common or noteworthy answers).
Lab A Sept. 28 (3 hr)	**— Instructor-led Discussion**: On Handout B with emphasis on Family and Social History including implications for treatment. **— Live Demonstration**: Construction of a family tree using guidelines in Handout B. **— Exercise**: Students practice constructing family trees; receive feedback. **— Exercise**: Students practice recording answers to family and social history questions from taped patient interviews; implications of each case discussed as feedback is given after each case.	Read **Handout C** (describing common complaints involving each organ system) Review "Systems Review" section of Handout B. Study sample **Decision Flow Chart** (giving questions to ask in exploring common chief complaints related to respiratory system)*

*Additional Decision Flowcharts will be provided later in course as part of each major organ system.

(Partial Syllabus, continued)

Date	Instructional Activities	Assignment for Next Session
Session 3 Oct. 1 (2 hr)	– **Mini-lecture:** Review Handout C stressing importance of systems review at all visits. – **Live Demonstration:** Use of Decision Flow Chart to explore hypothetical chief complaints & recording results on history form. – **Practice Interviews:** In pairs, using sample Flow Chart and patient scenarios, students explore chief complaints and record responses on form (instructor feedback).	**Exercise-to-be-handed-in:** Students list series of questions to explore specified chief complaints with additional complications (may use flowchart). Review parts of Handout B regarding recording data onto History forms.
Session 4 Oct. 3 (2 hr)	– **Live Demonstration:** Recording entire interview on History Form. – **Exercise:** Students record complete medical histories from audiotaped patient interviews. Class feedback and discussion.	Review all handouts to prepare for Lab B.
Lab B Oct. 5 (3 hr)	– **Practice Interviews:** In groups of three, students take complete histories from classmates primed with scenarios. Record interviews on audiotape; on replay, feedback from classmates and instructor.	Analyze incomplete case history forms and determine what additional questions should have been asked.
Session 5 Oct. 8 (2 hr)	– **Small Group Discussion:** In groups of four, students discuss assigned incomplete histories, focussing on how missing information could be important. – **Instructor-led Discussion:** Results of small group discussion compared with critical feedback. – **Practice Interviews:** In pairs and using patient scenarios, students take complete medical histories on History Form.	Prepare for Lab C and for Practical and Written exams.
Lab C (Any time during week)	– **Practice Interviews—Real Patients:** Assign each student to a pediatric resident. At mutual convenience during week, student obtains complete medical histories from parents of actual patients under care of resident. Feedback from resident.	Prepare for practical and written exams.
Session 6 Oct. 12 (3 hr)	– **Practical Exam:** Students take complete medical histories from primed classmates. (Terminal Competency for unit.) – **Written Exam:** Items sampling the intermediate competencies for unit.	

Index

other: B-3
Motion pictures, A-59/A-60, C-55, C-119, *C-130/C-133
Multiple-choice test, C-34
Multiple roles, B-6, B-7/B-8, B-9/B-10, B-11, B-16, B-19/B-20, B-23, B-25

Norm-referenced grading systems, C-29, *C-49/C-50, C-52
Normal curve, C-49/C-50

Objective examinations, C-29, *C-42/C-43
Objectives, A-29, A-31, A-33, A-37, A-47, A-50, B-9, B-24, B-25, B-132, B-136, C-94, C-95, C-105, C-113, C-114
Observation interview, A-21, C-5, *C-21/C-22
  see also Performance analysis, methods of
Observational reports, A-60, C-29, *C-38
Open-ended Question(naire):
  example: C-7
  other: C-6/C-7
Optimal professional performance:
  definition: A-10
  other: A-5, A-14, A-10/A-24, A-25, A-31
  see also Performance, professional
Oral examinations, C-29, *C-39
Overhead projection, B-133, C-55, C-119, *C-123/C-124

Panel of experts, *see* Group interview
Patient management problems, *see* Clinical simulations
Performance:
  definition: A-35
  other: A-47/A-48
   see also, Performance, professional; Performance, student
  Performance, professional:
   examples: B-75, B-110, B-123
   other: A-3, A-5/A-31, A-32, A-33/A-34, A-35/A-48, B-5/B-68, B-69, B-71/B-72, B-79/B-81, C-5/C-28
   see also Actual professional performance; Optimal professional performance
  performance student:
   examples: A-40/A-41, A-54, B-75, B-86, B-106, B-110, B-111, B-123, B-124
   other: A-37/A-38, A-43, A-45, A-46/A-48, A-52, A-55, A-71, A-72, B-70/B-81, B-82/B-87, B-97, B-100/B-112, B-132, B-136
   see also, Intermediate competencies
Performance analysis:
  definition: A-21
   See also specific methods, i.e.: Checklist; Critical incident technique; Group interview; Individual interview; Log diary; Observation interview; Questionnaire; Technical conference; Work participation
  other: A-20, A-22, A-24, A-25, A-26, A-29, A-31, B-56/B-61, B-62/B-68
  see also Performance analysis, methods of
  methods of: A-21/A-22, A-23, A-24, B-5, B-51/B-55, B-56/B-61, B-62/B-68, *C-5/C-28
Performance discrepancies:
  causes of, A-27/A-28
  definition: A-23
  example: A-28
  other: A-8, A-20/A-22, A-23, A-24, A-25/A-28, A-30, B-5, B-62/B-68
Performance standards, *definition:* A-26
Posttests:
  definition: A-44
  other: A-43/A-45, A-46, A-55, A-57, B-69, B-82, B-88/B-98, C-32, C-51, C-113
Practical examinations, A-59/A-60, C-29, *C-37
Prerequisite tests:
  definition: A-44
  other: A-43/A-45, A-46, A-55, A-57, B-69, B-82, B-88/B-98, C-32, C-113
Pretests:
  definition: A-44
  other: A-43/A-45, A-46, A-55, A-57, B-69, B-82, B-88/B-98, C-32, C-113
Problem-solving exercises, C-68
Professional competencies:

examples: B-75, B-110, B-123
other: A-35, A-37/A-38, A-40, A-41, A-52/53, A-72, B-70, B-71
see also Professional responsibility
Professional responsibility:
 definition: A-2
 examples: A-13, A-15
 other: A-5, A-9, A-12/A-13, A-14, A-17/A-18, A-25/A-31, A-33, A-37, B-5, B-12/B-15, B-16/B-25, B-42, B-46, B-48/B-49, B-56/B-61, B-71
Professional role:
 definition: A-11
 other: A-5, A-7, A-10, A-12, A-17, A-19, A-31, B-6/B-11, B-12/B-15, B-16/B-25, B-56/B-61
 see also Multiple roles
Professional setting, A-10, A-11, A-37, A-42, A-46
Programmed instruction, A-59, C-55, C-89, *C-97/C-112, C-115
 see also Linear Programmed instruction; Branching programmed instruction; and Traditional programmed instruction
Programmed lecture, B-133/B-134, C-54, *C-76/C-78
Progress test:
 definition: A-55
 other: A-57, C-31/C-32
Project assignments, A-60, C-29, *C-40
Providing a model:
 example: C-59
 other: A-59, C-56, *C-59/C-60

Questionnaire:
 examples: B-64/B-65, C-7
 other: A-21, A-22, C-5, *C-6/C-8, C-24, C-25, C-27
 see also Performance analysis, methods of

Real world experiences:
 example: C-71
 other: A-59, C-54, *C-71/C-72
Real world performance, *see* Performance, professional
Reinforcement, C-61/C-63
Reinforcing behavior:
 examples: C-62/C-63
 other: C-54, *C-61/C-63
Reliability, C-29, C-30, *C-33/C-35, C-51, C-53
Remedial instruction, A-43/A-45, A-55
Resources for simulation, A-32, A-38/A-39, *A-42, A-46, A-52, B-76
Responsibility, *see* Components (of a responsibility), Entire responsibility; and Professional responsibility
Role playing:
 example: C-66/C-67
 other: B-131, C-54
Role plays, A-59/A-60, C-9

Scope of responsibility, B-28, B-39, B-45/B-47, B-50
 see also Levels of detail
Score distribution:
 examples: B-89, B-91, B-93
 other: B-88, *B-89/B-90, B-91/B-92, B-93, C-51
 see also Histogram
Seating arrangements, B-143/B-144
Self-tests, A-55
Simulation, A-32/A-34, A-37/A-41, A-46, A-70, C-111
 see also Conditions, student; Highest level of simulation; Intermediate levels of simulation; Levels of simulation; and Resources for simulation
Simulation games:
 examples: C-69
 other: A-59/A-60, C-54, *C-68/C-70
Skill:
 definition: A-14

examples: A-15, B-41, B-43, B-44, B-76, B-109
  other: A-35/A-36, A-65, B-27/B-38, B-42, B-48
  see also Components (of a responsibility)
Slides, 35mm, A-59/A-60, B-131/B-135, C-55, C-76, C-97, *C-125/C-126
SME, *see* Subject matter experts
Software:
  definition: B-131
  other: B-132, B-136
Student competencies:
  example: A-62/A-64
  other: A-3, A-32/A-48, B-69/B-98, C-29/C-53
  see also Entry student competencies; Intermediate competencies; and Terminal student competencies
Student diagnosis, B-94/B-95, B-97/B-98
Student Progress, A-49, A-50, A-52, A-55, A-60/A-61, A-70
Student tutors, C-116/C-117
Subject matter experts, A-22, B-57, B-60/B-61, C-26
Survey course, B-16, B-21/B-22, B-23/B-24, B-25
Syllabus:
  examples: A-68/A-69, B-139/B-140
  other: A-49/A-51, A-60/A-61, *A-66/A-69, A-70/A-72, B-99, B-137/B-141
Symmetrical curve, *see* Normal curve

Task analysis, C-21/C-22, C-24, C-27
Teaching assistants, C-54, *C-93, C-116
Teaching observations, A-55
Technical conference, A-21, C-5, *C-26
  see also Performance analysis, methods of
Terminal student competency:
  definition: A-33
  examples: A-42, B-75, B-110, B-123
  other: A-34, A-35/A-48, A-50/A-51, A-52, A-53, A-55, A-57, A-61, A-66, A-70, A-72, B-69/B-81, B-130,
    B-132, B-133, B-134/B-135
  see also Highest level of simulation
Tests, A-43/A-45, A-55/A-56, C-30/C-35
  see also Pretests; Progress tests; Posttests; Prerequisite tests; and Evaluation
Traditional programmed instruction, C-97, C-105, C-106
Transmitting information, A-65, A-67, C-54, C-56, *C-57/C-58, C-98
Transparencies, *see* Overhead projection
Trigger films, A-59, C-54, *C-85/C-88

Unit of instruction:
  definition: A-50
  examples: A-62/A-64, B-127/B-128
  other: A-50/A-53, A-57/A-65, A-66/A-67, A-70/A-72, B-93, B-113, B-118/B-129, B-134/B-135, C-115/C-117

Validity, C-29, C-30, *C-33/C-35, C-53
Videotape recordings, A-59/A-60, B-131/B-135, C-55, C-98, C-115/C-116, *C-134/C-136

Work participation, A-21, C-5, *C-23
  see also Performance analysis, methods of